wild
MEDITERRANEAN

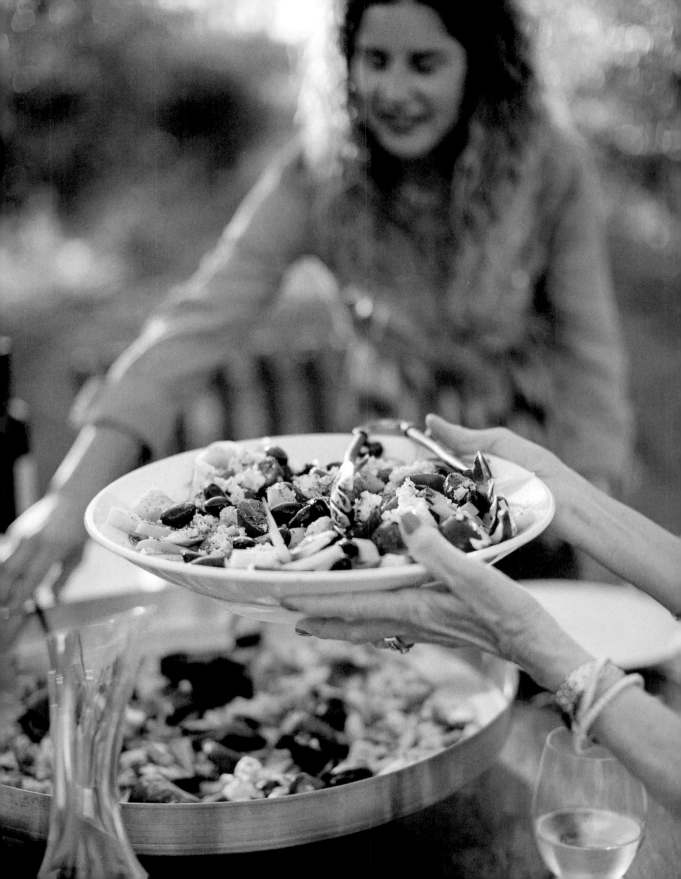

wild MEDITERRANEAN

THE AGE-OLD, SCIENCE-NEW PLAN FOR A HEALTHY GUT, WITH FOOD YOU CAN TRUST

STELLA METSOVAS

PAM KRAUSS BOOKS/ AVERY

New York

Pam Krauss Books / Avery
an imprint of Penguin Random House LLC
375 Hudson Street
New York, New York 10014

Most Avery books are available at special quantity discounts
for bulk purchase for sales promotions, premiums, fund-
raising, and educational needs. Special books or book excerpts
also can be created to fit specific needs. For details, write
SpecialMarkets@penguinrandomhouse.com.

Library of Congress Cataloging-in-Publication Data

Names: Metsovas, Stella, author.
Title: Wild Mediterranean : the age-old, science-new plan for a
healthy gut, with food you can trust / Stella Metsovas.
Description: New York : Pam Krauss/Avery, [2017]
Identifiers: LCCN 2016059049 | ISBN 9780553496468
(hardback)
Subjects: LCSH: Gastrointestinal system—Microbiology. |
Nutrition. | Digestion. | Diet—Mediterranean Region. |
Self-care, Health. | BISAC: HEALTH & FITNESS /
Healthy Living. | COOKING / Regional & Ethnic /
Mediterranean.
Classification: LCC QR171.G29 M487 2017 |
DDC 612.3/2—dc23
LC record available at https://lccn.loc.gov/2016059049
p.   cm.

Printed in the United States of America
10 9 8 7 6 5 4 3 2 1

Book design by Ashley Tucker

The recipes contained in this book are to be followed exactly
as written. The publisher is not responsible for your specific
allergy needs that may require medical supervision. The
publisher is not responsible for any adverse reactions to the
recipes contained in this book.

To my husband, Steve,
may we always live
happily ever after in our village.

CONTENTS

PREFACE: WILD TIMES 9

introduction: Why Wild Is Better 16

chapter 1: Your Forgotten Organ 25

chapter 2: The Wild Detox: Re-wilding Your Body with Whole Foods 38

chapter 3: The Wild Kitchen 78

chapter 4: Village-to-Table Recipes 94

chapter 5: How to Live Wild 182

CONCLUSION 207

RESOURCES 209

ACKNOWLEDGMENTS 211

NOTES 212

INDEX 217

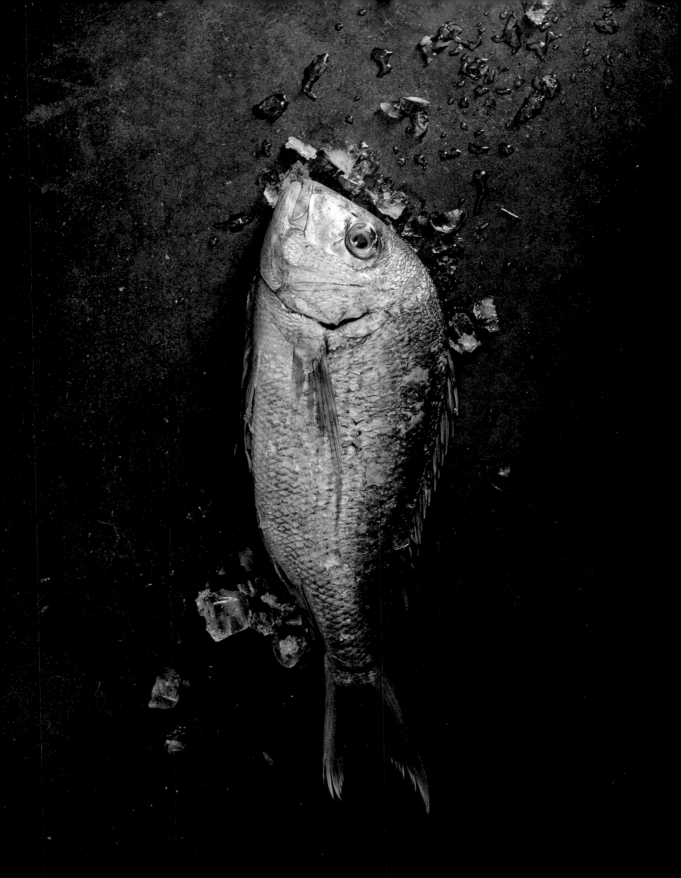

WILD TIMES

I GREW UP WILD.

When I was just three years old, my beloved grandfather, Constantine, decided it was time for me to learn how to fish. My family and I were visiting my paternal grandparents at their cottage in the ancient village of Methana, on the southern Peloponnese Greek peninsula made up of steep, rocky slopes. He whisked me off in his *kaiki*, one of the brightly colored traditional fishing boats found in the Mediterranean waters surrounding the Greek Islands. We finally stopped at one of his lucky fishing spots, where he showed me his favorite maneuvers, using just a simple pole. I was so thrilled when the first little fish landed on my line. My grandfather helped me pull the flipping, shiny guy into the boat.

Back at my grandparents' house, my grandfather introduced me to the sometimes messy reality of wild food. Looking rather pleased with myself, I held the gutted, raw fish as he snapped a photo. It was a proud moment for him, too. He was teaching me how to harvest and prepare food that came directly from the sea surrounding us, the same way he'd been taught by his mother and father, and they had been by theirs. I'd solidified my bond with nature, and I embraced a pastime that had been practiced in this part of the world for centuries. Somehow I think I sensed the importance of this event—that I'd completed one of the critical first rites of growing up the "Wild Mediterranean" way, or a way of living that's rooted deeply in age-old tradition, our natural surroundings, and the close-knit bond of a community.

Looking back, it occurs to me that many of my early memories involve food in some way. In my grandparents' sun-bathed hamlet, the villagers threw huge parties known as *panagiria* in the center of their small towns each spring and summer—open-air events filled with great food, local wine, and music to entice people of every age to take part in the customary Greek dances. The men would roast lambs and chickens on huge fire spits, and the women would make their specialty dishes from the bountiful produce of the season, such as spinach and feta pies, *yemista* (stuffed vegetables), and *horiatiki* (village salad) served with *psomi* (stone-baked bread). I recall tables laden with desserts, from honey-laced baklava to custard-filled *galaktoboureko* to mounds of curiously fluffy-yet-crunchy *koulourakia*, Greek Easter cookies.

> Beyond the food, there was real connection among the people. They delighted in the wildness of the landscape that surrounded them.

Beyond the food, there was real connection among the people. These villagers shared everything from the joy of birth to the grief of death. They delighted in the wildness of the landscape that surrounded them and spent time walking and hiking the volcanic hills, fishing and swimming in the blue waters. Nearly everyone kept a garden and tended olive and citrus trees, pressing their own oil and juices. These happy pursuits never stopped, even in old age.

My parents carried this way of life with them when they settled in southern California. As a result, I was always a little different from other kids. If you've seen the film *My Big Fat Greek Wedding*, then you've got some idea. Few California girls were named Stella—at least not in the mid-1990s—and my parents had strong ideas of how a young woman should be raised: knee-length (or longer) dresses and no makeup (although my mom did slip me some lip gloss behind my father's back). My brother and I were not allowed to stay indoors and watch TV when it was sunny outside, which in southern California was pretty much all the time. Invariably, our parents shooed us outside to play, and encouraged us to run, swim, climb trees, and explore on our own. After all, that's how *they* were raised.

They carried on other traditions in California, too. When my father's friends and family moved from Athens to the US, he emulated the big village parties by inviting everyone to our house for huge feasts. These boisterous affairs often went on late into the night as dozens of cousins, aunts, uncles, friends, and neighbors would descend with Mediterranean specialties. Only the music changed. In addition to Greek standards, my parents played everything from Michael Jackson to classic rock 'n roll. The rest of the revelry remained the same: They would drink wine, sing loudly, dance with abandon, and talk for hours. But above all, they would eat—lamb roasted with oregano and potatoes, a medley of bright peppers sprinkled with feta, stuffed grape leaves. One of my favorite dishes was *briam*, perfectly ripe seasonal vegetables baked in olive oil. It's a simple-sounding dish, but it takes skill to get just right.

Our everyday cooking also illustrated my family's Mediterranean ways. My mother balked at packaged fare, and fast food was out of the question. We ate dishes such as braised pastured meats slowly cooked in earthenware, beans baked with tomatoes and herbs, and stews made according to season. She packed moussaka for school lunch. Longing for a taste of home, my mother continued to make some of the hearty specialty dishes for my father, even if it required ingenuity on her part to find the right ingredients. Let's just say my parents were among the few people in southern California who knew how to source a whole lamb when needed.

As kids, we returned to Greece each summer. Even though my brother and I often were groggy following the international flight, we could barely contain ourselves during the two-hour ride from Athens to the familiar sights and sounds of Methana. Within moments, he and I

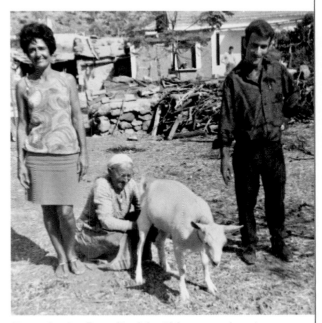

My grandmother, Evangeline, left, with her aunt and cousin in our village, Methana, Greece.

stepped back into a slower rhythm of life. We chatted easily with the villagers we'd known all our lives. After breakfast each morning, my grandmother would give us a bit of money and we'd head out on our bikes, picking up a few snacks and little games at the small store near my grandparents' house. In California, we still ate pretty "wild" in comparison to other families, but we would still get the occasional processed treat. In my grandparents' village, good luck if you want a candy bar! Well into the 1990s, there was just one brand of chips and two options for ice cream. The only classic Western staple was Coca-Cola.

When we brought these "delicacies" home, our relatives would moan, clutch their hearts, and complain with such vigor that you'd think the world was ending. Once, my aunt dramatically shook her hands to the heavens as she wailed, tears in her eyes, "Why, Stella! Why do you buy these fake things? Why, when we have fresh peaches from your uncle's tree or Maria's *koulourakia*? Why?!"

Aside from the occasional store-bought treat, though, we were raised eating the way the people in my parents' village have for centuries, and that—along with fortunate genetics— ensured that we grew up strong, tall, and lean. By age ten, I was already five feet five inches tall, with a long torso and long legs. I had shiny hair past my shoulders and clear skin. I slept well and felt great. I couldn't have been any healthier.

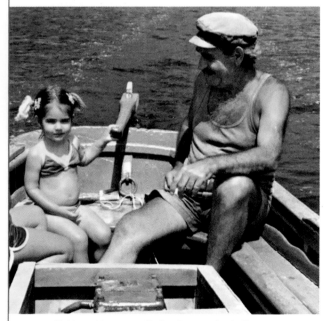

Fishing with my grandfather Constantine in Greece.

When I was ten years old and swimming at a public pool near our home in Orange County, California, a coach asked my mother if I'd considered swimming competitively.

"She's a natural," he told my mom.

As it turned out, he was right. Within months, I was one of the youngest swimmers in advanced leagues. By age eleven—just one year after starting my training—I was competing in the Junior Olympics on the USA Swimming circuit.

I awoke before dawn to swim and

then returned to the pool for hours of after-school training. I spent a good chunk of my life looking down at the blurry blue bottom of a pool. Like thousands of kids across the country, I trained to compete at the highest levels. For a while Olympic medalist Janet Evans trained in her own lane at the end of the same pool as I did, and I would sometimes catch a glimpse of her. I believed that if I worked hard, maybe someday I'd stand on a podium with three gold medals, just as Janet had. I'm thankful for the stringent work ethic competitive swimming imparted to me. It shaped the way I approach life, even now.

But the training took its toll, and not in a way that you'd expect.

My mother followed the coach's instruction and shifted what I ate to a hyper-low-fat/high-carbohydrate diet, the recommended regimen for young athletes at that time and still followed by many to this day. The reasoning: Fats are bad, carbs provide fuel. For some people, this diet might not have been much of a change. For me, though, it was a radical departure from the olive-oiled, meat-and-fish-filled, vegetable-packed world of Mediterranean fare that I'd thrived on growing up. I went from regular meals of lean proteins, seasonal vegetables, and occasional grilled lamb to heaping plates of pasta, protein bars, and coach-approved sugar-laden sports drinks. Olive oil—an evil fat—was a no-no.

Something changed in me. My hair started falling out. At first, we blamed the chlorine, but then I started succumbing to colds and flus regularly, although I had rarely been sick as a child. My olive complexion turned pale. I had no energy. I was constantly fatigued, listless, and bloated. I looked nothing like the sun-kissed Mediterranean girl I'd been just a couple of years earlier. But in competitive training, you don't take days off. Part of the program is learning to push through obstacles, whether they're mental or physical.

So I pushed and pushed until one day, I just snapped and decided to quit.

Abandoning a routine that involved hard physical exercise several hours a day added a layer of depression to my overall lethargy. I later read that Olympic swimmer Michael Phelps also felt depressed when he gave up his intensive training routine, but at the time I didn't know what was happening to me. I just felt terrible.

My mother took me to doctors, who couldn't figure out what was wrong. One diagnosed me with severe anemia, although he couldn't explain why an active teenager with no discernible health issues would develop such a serious condition.

By the time I headed off for my freshman year of college I was back to eating better but continued on a steady diet of protein bars and sugar-laden granola, and my health complaints continued unabated. Determined to understand why my life had changed so drastically, I considered two possible majors at school: sports medicine or nutrition sciences. When a counselor explained that majoring in nutrition involved a deep knowledge of food and how it interacts with the body, I was sold.

Fascinated by the subject, I lived and breathed nutrition. For years, I relied on the conventional wisdom I was taught in school: Weight loss was simply a matter of calories in, calories out. I even became a vegan, rigorously, and often joylessly, trying to choke down all the prescribed macro- and micronutrients each day. Yet I still didn't feel completely healed.

After graduation, I started a nutrition consulting business in Southern California, meeting day after day with clients whose complaints and conditions were eerily similar to the ones I'd experienced when I was younger. Although many of them wanted to lose weight, they also reported other issues such as lack of energy, bloating, depression, and cloudy thinking. I could certainly empathize. Even as I treated my clients, I was dragging *myself* through the day. I wasn't as depleted as I had been when I was an anemic teenager and training six hours a day in a swimming pool, but I wasn't exactly pulsing with energy, either. I needed a jolt of caffeine to kick myself into gear each morning, I fell into a slump most afternoons, and I had a tough time getting to sleep and staying asleep. I also found it difficult to deal with the common day-to-day stressors and often felt blue or anxious. My elimination was irregular, and, like many of us, I was also struggling to be consistent with workouts and maintain a lean frame. Plus, I had headaches and cravings, especially for oily pizza around the time of my period. I was still grappling with a slight case of anemia. Still, because the symptoms weren't dramatic, I accepted the low hum of my life, as most of us do.

One particularly challenging day, I thought about the photo of me with my gutted fish. It occurred to me that the people I know who lived in Greece never had such symptoms. I know this because village life encourages sharing just about everything, including health issues—right down to one's bowel movements (!) and the smallest aches and pains. Understanding and discussing the natural functions of our bodies is part of how that community shares. So it gnawed at me that the Mediterranean villagers remained robust and healthy well into old age while relatively young people came into my office with such a wide variety of complaints.

It took me years to discover the connection between health, longevity, and the food we eat—specifically, how that food affects the landscape of the digestive system, from which so much of our vigor, immunity, and wellness emanates—but when I did, it challenged everything that I had been taught, by both my teachers and other experts in the nutrition field. I realized that I needed to go back to the beginning, back to where my own health and vibrancy came from. I needed to rediscover the lessons that my mother and father and their families and generations of families before them had taught me. I needed to reconnect with the whole, wild Mediterranean foods that nourished my body and the community spirit that fed my soul. I had to, in every sense of the world, find my "wild" again.

If you're reading this book, then I'm willing to guess that somewhere along the way you too lost your native self. Maybe you don't have as much energy as you think you should, you can't maintain a healthy weight, or you're battling chronic illness. Maybe it just feels like your "light" isn't shining so brightly. Whatever your concerns might be, you'll be relieved to know that most if not all of these maladies stem from a single source: a digestive system that's sorely in need of repair and rejuvenation. It's very likely that your gut—the hub of digestive health—isn't getting the "wild" or whole-food–based, living nutrition it needs to thrive, and in turn, keep all of your body's systems working optimally. With this book, I'm going to help you connect with your own wild roots in the spirit of healing and staying healthy. I'll share the traditional wisdom— from eating habits to daily rituals—that is the key to living a long, satisfying, *well* life. (Not to mention the science that completely supports it!) So please join me on this journey back to where I come from, where my people come from, and where, ultimately, better lives are made. Welcome to the Wild Mediterranean.

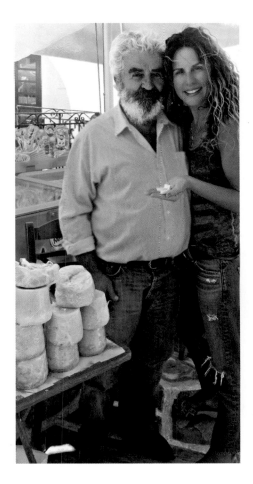

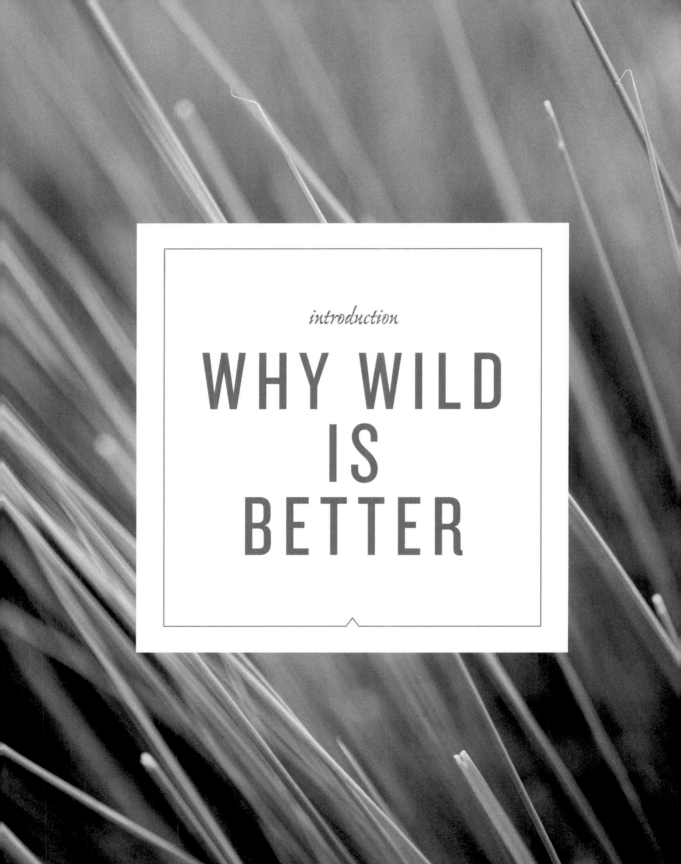

WHY WILD IS BETTER

"A village means that you are not alone,
knowing that in the people, the trees, the earth,
there is something that belongs to you,
waiting for you when you are not there."

Cesare Pavese

PEOPLE ARE WILLING TO TRY *ANYTHING* TO FEEL BETTER. WE SPEND BILLIONS OF DOLLARS ON designer vitamins and minerals, heart-pumping exercise programs, body-relaxing yoga, mind-calming meditation retreats, and fancy five-star spas. We fill our shopping carts with heirloom vegetables and so-called miracle grains, and pour money into the latest super, energy-boosting elixirs, green juices, and smoothies. We're even willing to chew on hemp and chia seeds and follow ultrastrict detox diets, fasts, and cleanses. *And yet*, we're still sick, tired, overweight, superstressed, and unhappy. In the US alone, 60 to 70 million people suffer from digestive diseases such as gastroesophageal reflux, ulcers, Crohn's disease, celiac disease, colitis, and irritable bowel syndrome—which often are entry points for other illnesses. Even if we don't necessarily see ourselves as sick, we're still throwing back a staggering number of diet pills, sleeping medications, antidepressants, painkillers, and antacids. Maybe—just maybe—it has something to do with the mountains of sugar and piles of processed foods that we eat every day, despite the numerous admonitions from nutrition experts that these things are a danger to our health. *Why, despite all the health advice—from the experts on down to Instagram "celebrities" offering so-called solutions—are we still eating like crazy and feeling run-down and sick?*

Well, what if I told you that you could change all that? And that it was as simple and straightforward as following the diet and lifestyle choices that are still practiced today in the

Mediterranean, a lifestyle that has evolved over centuries to nurture and support healthy digestion and a thriving microbiome?

Take these two modern examples of Wild Mediterranean life, both closely resembling people I know:

George is a handsome goat herder in his early fifties who lives in the Greek Peloponnese area of Sparta. He's lean and strong—which indicates that he has a healthy amount of testosterone—plus he has a zest for life. Each morning, he starts his day early with a shot of olive oil and a piece of high-fiber barley husk bread topped with some feta cheese. (A paltry breakfast by Western standards but actually the optimal combination of fat and carbohydrates to sustain the body!) He follows his goats around the rocky landscape for a few hours as they eat fresh grass and herbs, until early afternoon, when he leads them all back home. Lunch is the biggest meal of the day and consists of abundant amounts of roasted vegetables, a bit of braised lamb, lentil soup, and/or boiled greens served with lemon and olive oil. After lunch, he likes to "spend a little time" with his wife, the local euphemism for a common ritual of having post-lunch sex. Afterward, he heads back out with his goats until about six p.m., when he either gets together with friends or spends time with his two children. Then it's off to bed, where he makes sure to get plenty of sleep each night.

Then there's Sophia, a beautiful young woman in her early thirties who lives in a small seaside town not far from Florence, Italy. Sophia is college-educated and works full-time in an advertising agency. With a lithe figure, flawless skin, and lovely long hair, she is the image of health. Even though her desk job requires that she sit for much of the day, her daily life still includes a

Eating delicious, whole foods + moving the way nature originally intended us to + connecting with other like-minded people = your best health.

No "superfoods," magic potions, or strict deprivation regimens are required. I know that it sounds too good to be true—and way too easy. But I've seen the miraculous effects of this approach firsthand.

lot of natural, active movement, especially walking—whether it's to work, to the market, or to see friends—and a healthy work-life balance. On Sundays she shops at the local farmers' market and stocks up on kitchen essentials: small fish such as sardines (which she's been eating since she was a small child) and a wide array of seasonal fruits and vegetables. When she isn't cooking for friends and family, she prepares simple meals for herself.

Both Sophia and George are examples of a healthy, well-rounded life. While I'm not suggesting that you won't reap the benefits of this program

> I discovered that a diet made up of foods traditionally found in the Mediterranean (lean meat, seafood, seasonal fruits and vegetables, olive oil, and other healthy fats) provides the optimal balance of nutrients to keep the gut—the engine responsible for powering our bodies and immune system—running the way it should.

if you don't acquire a herd of goats or move to a remote Mediterranean village, do consider how George and Sophia approach their daily routines—with balance and a focus on wholesome foods that nourish all the body's systems (specifically the digestive system, or the gut, which we'll talk much more about in a bit), natural movement, and socializing. You, too, could benefit from this simple equation:

Eating delicious, whole foods + moving the way nature originally intended us to + connecting with other like-minded people = your best health.

No "superfoods," magic potions, or strict deprivation regimens are required. I know that it sounds too good to be true—and way too easy. But I've seen the miraculous effects of this approach firsthand. In addition to traveling around the globe to villages in places like Peru, Norway, France, Spain, and Mexico to collect the lifestyle secrets of the longest-living among them, I've also spent every summer since I was born in my native Greece. In these villages, chronic diseases—especially those linked to poor digestive health—are virtually nonexistent and life expectancies of ninety to one hundred years (and older) are *common*. Within these remote corners of the world, people have mastered the art of living: actively and happily. And it hasn't stressed their bodies, their budgets, or their psyches to do so. When I brought these concepts to my practice, I successfully nurtured my clients back to vibrancy, wellness, and joy. And along the way I found my own path to good health.

I discovered that a diet made up of foods traditionally found in the Mediterranean (lean meat, seafood, seasonal fruits and vegetables, olive oil, and other healthy fats) provides the optimal balance of nutrients to keep the gut—the engine responsible for powering our bodies and immune system—running the way it should. It's now thought that the microbiome acts as a "second genome" to our DNA sequencing, meaning if our DNA is the blueprint that dictates how prone we are to disease, the microbiome is the overlay to that blueprint that can either flip the switch for less-than-ideal health conditions or keep them at bay. As you'll learn in Chapter 2, a healthy gut is the secret to resolving chronic conditions like asthma, eczema, depression, and acne; treating diseases such as heart disease, high blood pressure, diabetes, and cancer; not to mention maintaining a healthy, lean weight (thanks to an efficiently fueled metabolism) and living a long, ailment-free life.

Let's make one thing clear from the start: This is *not* a diet book. Well, at least not in the sense that the primary and ultimate goal of my methods is to result in weight loss complete with dogmatic do's and don'ts, calorie-counting, and macronutrient policing (carbs bad! fat bad!). Rather—like most of the advice in this book—I'm taking things back to the roots, including the very notion of "diet." The term derives from the Greek word *diaita*, meaning "way of life, regimen, and dwelling." And that's exactly what this book is: a guide to regaining your health and digestive balance by making a series of long-lasting lifestyle choices, from approaching the world with childlike curiosity and a sense of play, to regularly enjoying nature, to minimizing stress and getting better-quality sleep (and more of it), to using self-care products that keep you feeling beautiful from the outside in. I call this approach Wild Mediterranean not only because all the principles are based on the successful health practices and foods favored in that part of the world, but also because getting "wild"—or aligning yourself more closely with nature, from your food to your surroundings—is essential for building optimal health. Or more specifically, a resilient, robust digestive system.

Many of my clients come to me looking for an easy fix, whether they want to lose weight or remedy a chronic condition. I always tell them that there's no magic solution. I do, however, know that the process of restoring your digestive health can also bring you to a profound, meaningful connection with yourself, your surroundings, and those around you.

On a deep, perhaps subconscious, level, Wild Mediterranean living resonates within us because it's connecting us with a community through food and culture, whether or not we're actually from this particular part of the world. It's connecting us to somewhere we've been, where we are now, or where we'd like ultimately to be. Unlike the Paleo approach, which asks followers to connect to their caveman forebears, who were slurping up bugs and clubbing animals to death (though, to be fair, they also weren't eating processed food), connecting to this "food tribe"—along with the delicious traditional foods that nurture digestive health—is relatable. We can all envision ourselves as—and aspire to be—members of a thriving, close-knit community where health is synonymous with living joyfully, whether we live in a bustling urban neighborhood or a sparsely populated rural area. And you can achieve it, too. It all starts with adopting a new diaita—or way of living.

> True wellness begins with proper digestive health.

To begin, we'll talk about your body and how it operates. True wellness begins with proper digestive health. I'll walk you through how this system works, why it makes the difference between chronic disease and longevity, and signs that yours might not be performing as it should. Then I'll outline exactly how we're going to create and maintain optimal digestive health, beginning with a biome-healing "pre-tox" followed by a three-day whole-food detox that's specifically designed to suit your unique health issues and to reestablish digestive balance. We'll talk about the delicious new go-to foods that will rejuvenate and support your body, and I'll outline a plan for enjoying these foods every day, all year long. You'll see that there's no need to feel deprived on the path to health. The only thing I'm going to take away is your discomfort and discontent, and in exchange you'll get a long, healthy life fueled by a wide spectrum of versatile, satisfying foods that will in turn promote a greater diversity of microbes in your gut.

To help you get a head start on your new lifestyle—and help you continue to support your digestive health—you'll find fifty of my favorite recipes inspired by the cuisines of Greece, Spain, France, and Italy. I've taken classic staples like roast chicken and given them a

"Four Countries: Four Ways" spin. For example, the same basic technique can take you from paprika-peppered Spain, to the signature lemon and oregano of Greece, to the lavender-scented herbes de Provence of France, to the rosemary and sun-dried tomato notes of Italy. (Because no one ever said it needs to be all Greek, all the time.) These foods aren't just delicious, they're scientifically proven to keep your digestive health in balance owing to their beneficially "wild" nature (something we'll talk much more about in the next chapter). I'll help you "wild" your pantry and fridge with shopping lists and must-have staples, along with plenty of kitchen tips and tricks to guide you through the cooking process.

From there we'll turn our focus to living wild, or boosting health with other simple lifestyle changes inspired by my Mediterranean forebears and scientifically proven to support strong digestive health. This includes a daily exercise plan (no need for the gym or scheduled classes!), stress relief techniques, ways to create a closer community, or how to find your own village. After all, it takes a village to stay healthy! I'll also throw in some of my favorite natural beauty secrets for keeping your hair shiny and skin radiant using age-old wisdom and Wild Mediterranean ingredients.

Ultimately, I created the Wild Mediterranean program because I wanted to protect people from the inaccuracies that are so pervasive in the health and diet world and give my clients the tools for long-term success. I was tired of seeing my clients, who after months of hard work on calorie-centric diets or juice cleanses, would end up at their starting weight, if not heavier. From that frustration came the resolve to give people access to what I've come to know as a health expert. I've seen the data that supports what Mediterranean cultures have known for centuries: that eating certain nutrient-dense foods combined with living a life full of natural movement, joy, and community leads to long-standing health, especially in the gut. Couple that with the emerging science of just how crucial our digestive health is to overall wellness, and we have a clear picture of how we can finally succeed in losing weight, beating chronic illness, and generally feeling better. And the best part? If you fall off the path, you can always come back. There are no absolutes here; only the requirement that you have a sense of adventure, the belief that change is good, and the knowledge that true wellness is in your hands.

Kalí órexi! (Good appetite!)

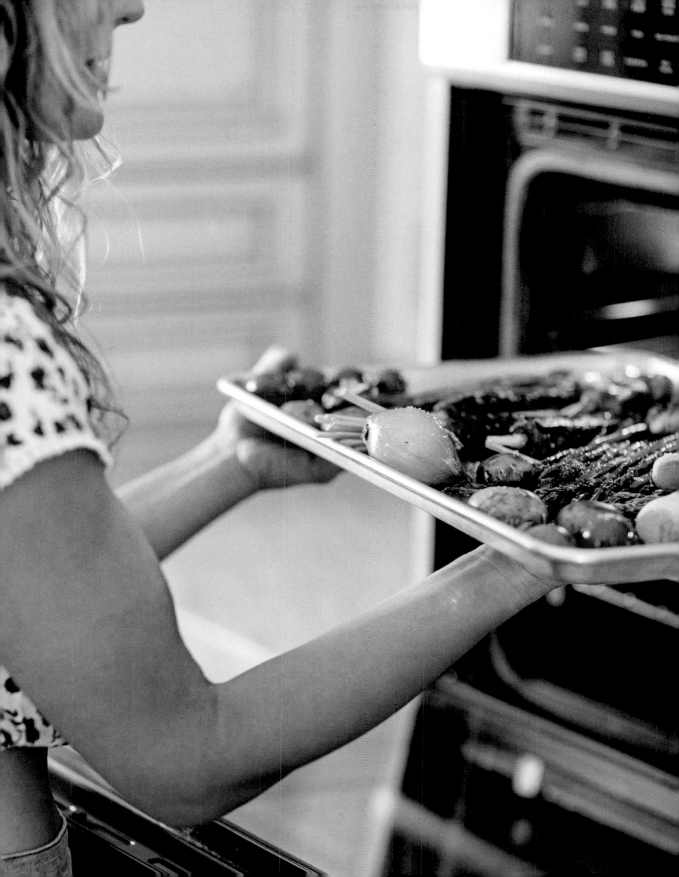

chapter 1

YOUR FORGOTTEN ORGAN

Understanding the Gut and Why It Matters to Your Health

> "Everything has been said before,
> but since nobody listens we have to keep
> going back and beginning all over again."
>
> André Gide

> "All disease begins in the gut."
>
> Hippocrates

FROM THE TIME I STARTED WORKING AS A NUTRITIONIST, MY CLIENTS CAME TO ME WITH A WIDE range of complaints: everything from sluggish metabolism and excessive weight, to fatigue, headaches, and mood swings, to digestive discomfort and skin issues, to chronic conditions like type 2 diabetes, arthritis, and high blood pressure. I'd counsel them through their individual maladies, but I never saw a connection among all these cases until the day I took "the test."

In 2007, I attended a digestive health seminar sponsored by one of the largest laboratory testing facilities in the world. At its conclusion, everyone was handed a test, known as a GI panel kit, which helps identify issues in the gut. Up until that point, my only understanding of the gut was pretty much input/output. After all, this test had traditionally been used pretty narrowly to diagnose digestive disorders like Crohn's disease or diverticulitis. When I returned to my office, I tucked the kit into the back of a file cabinet. After all, I felt *fine* . . . not amazing, but I didn't have any symptoms of being "sick." I chalked up feeling run-down and depleted to being busy, running a successful practice, and maybe not getting as much sleep as I needed.

Months later, I stumbled across the test. It was close to its expiration date, so I thought, *Why not take it before it's too late?*

The results left me thunderstruck. The report showed a disproportionate level of bacteria and the presence of microbial pathogens in my gut, which meant I was inadequately absorbing micronutrients such as iron and basic cell-building essentials like protein and fats.

I recalled a swim meet in Santa Barbara, where I'd finished a 200-meter heat, gotten out of the pool, and nearly passed out on the ground next to the starting blocks. My mother panicked, but my coach dismissed it as meet-related stress. A blood test and GI panel told the real story: I had abnormally low levels of ferritin—the protein that stores and controls the amount of iron in the body. Apparently I wasn't absorbing it properly, thanks to small intestinal bacterial overgrowth. I finally had the answer to my "unexplained" severe anemia. I wanted to call my old swim coach and say, "Here's the reason I couldn't push myself any harder!"

> It struck me that the foundation of health lay in the gut, the forgotten organ. As Hippocrates intuited some two thousand years before me, I recognized that the gut was the key to developing a new program for my clients.

These findings prompted me to dig deeper and learn more about why something seemingly isolated in my gut could have such far-reaching health repercussions. I eventually learned that all of this had started years earlier, beginning with the coach, doctor, and nutritionist-prescribed "athlete's diet." Add to that intense physical training, and I'd created the perfect storm for a condition that was depriving my system of nutrients and throwing my internal systems into complete disarray. Despite following all the "golden rules" of nutrition, this imbalance went untreated for years and became more severe over time. Even though I was an adult—and a nutritionist at that—I called my mother in tears. The mystery illness I'd suffered as a teen had never gone away.

But then my athlete's never-give-in mentality kicked in, and I was motivated to find a solution. And not just for me—for my clients, too. I read everything about digestive health I could find. I attended dozens of professional conferences on cutting-edge subjects such as nutrigenomics, the study of the effects of food and nutrition on gene expression. (That's right—you are more than your hereditary destiny!) The more I learned, the more I saw a common thread through most, if not all, of my clients' cases: poor digestive health. It struck me that the foundation of health lay in the gut, the forgotten organ that has long been written off as the collection spot for food eaten and poop-to-be. As Hippocrates intuited some two thousand years before me, I recognized that the gut was the key to developing a new program for my clients.

Of course nutritionists, researchers, scientists, and health experts are all looking at the gut now, but up to 2000 they were just starting to focus on the microbiome; by 2015 there were nearly twelve thousand studies published on the subject. Among them were experiments dedicated to exploring the link between microbial imbalance and the immune system; and all of the research confirmed the relationship between poor diet and a range of health disorders, including infertility, coronary disease, diabetes, and even cancer. And you know you're really on to something when Silicon Valley gets involved. A genomic research company called uBiome wants to do for the microbiome what earlier researchers did for DNA. Working in collaboration with the CDC, uBiome plans to analyze a large number of stool samples to help "sequence" the modern microbiome. Part of uBiome's long-term plan is to develop a Microbiome Disruption Index to track how factors like antibiotics, foods, lifestyle, and stress can alter the gut and hamper key functions, particularly the immune system. They also plan to explore how our microbiomes can be shifted and reshaped to potentially benefit generations to come.

These advancements in microbiome sequencing technology helped me understand how you not only can feed beneficial gut bacteria, but can also quantitatively verify how this daily healthful practice affects overall health. This rich pool of data has helped me develop and hone a program that would allow my clients to heal their guts and restore optimal health not only to their digestive systems, but to their entire body.

It all starts with what we eat and how we live, and it turns out that the best practices for optimal digestive health aren't cutting-edge, or even new for that matter. They're the very same foods and traditions that my ancestors have observed in the Mediterranean for generations. These "wild" ingredients and lifestyle observances help the microbiome thrive and, in turn, support overall health because of how they nurture the colonies of beneficial bacteria in our gut.

Your Internal Ecosystem

We commonly refer to the gut in positive ways. He's got guts. I have a gut feeling. Yet, we rarely consider how the state of our digestive tract can impact our overall lives—and we rarely discuss the state of our own gut in polite company. But the human gut is a true wonder. It harbors a dynamic, complex microbial environment known as the microbiome. An average human gut is host to more than two pounds of bacteria, just a bit less than the weight of a human brain. You most likely know that your gut digests food; but here's something I'll bet you didn't know: More than *70 percent* of the body's immune system tissues reside in this metabolic organ. This portion of the immune system is referred to as gut-associated lymphoid tissue (GALT). These lymphatic cells are some of your body's most vigorous defenders, developing antibodies to combat invading microorganisms. These little guys work tirelessly without fanfare to protect you every moment of the day. But when your gut and all its beneficial bacteria fall out of balance—most likely from an overgrowth of harmful bacteria or pathogens—that work is disrupted. The good bacteria become overwhelmed trying to chase after what they perceive to be a constant stream of offenders. As a result, your immune system's first line of defense gets run-down, leaving you vulnerable to disease.

Also living in our guts are toll-like receptors (TLRs). These respond to the presence of unknown antigens—or suspected bad guys—by unleashing an inflammatory response to what they perceive as infection in the gut. Believe it or not, this inflammation isn't a bad thing. In fact, a little bit of inflammation, when it comes to fighting off infection, is good. It stimulates damaged tissues to heal. However, it is possible to have too much of a good thing. Some foods—like processed products, sugar, and dairy—possess antigens that trigger the immune system to produce antibodies against them. While all foods contain potentially antigenic molecules—and any of these can trigger an immunogenic reaction—some foods, such as the ones listed above, are more common offenders than others. Eating these foods regularly can put your body in a constant state of inflammation. Even more alarmingly, some processed foods can fool the TLRs into thinking they're good guys. So if your system doesn't send out a hostile greeting team—either because it doesn't know any better or it's too taxed from dealing with all the other antigen action—then these potentially dangerous molecules get a free ride in your system. That's why when the gut's ecosystem is disrupted, the result is often inflammatory diseases such as rheumatoid arthritis, gastroesophageal reflux disease (GERD), lupus, fibromyalgia, multiple sclerosis, Hashimoto's thyroiditis, psoriasis, inflammatory bowel disease (IBD), and pelvic inflammatory disease (PID).

Dysbiosis and You

In nature—and in health—symbiosis, different organisms existing together in harmony, is crucial. This balanced state is what's considered eubiotic, 'eu" from the Greek word for "good" or "healthy," and "bios" meaning "life." As we've learned from nature, when a delicate ecosystem is thrown out of this balance, chaos ensues. If a natural predator is eliminated, populations of their natural prey explode. A similar concept is at work in your gut. If whole colonies of damaging microbes are left unchecked, they will eventually overwhelm the beneficial ones. In turn, organisms that are not usually predominant in our intestines, such as over-populated strains of unfriendly bacteria, yeast, and protozoa, can take charge. Thus starts a vicious cycle that can make the imbalance even greater. The result is called dysbiosis, and its impact

> As we've learned from nature, when a delicate ecosystem is thrown out of this balance, chaos ensues. A similar concept is at work in your gut.

on the body is far-reaching, though it doesn't affect everyone the same way. Problems stemming from dysbiosis can range from mild to extremely debilitating, depending on the extent of the gut's bacterial imbalance. It can alter how your brain functions—causing anything from "cloudy" thinking to emotional fluctuation—and has even been connected to psychiatric disorders, including depression. Scientists have found that dysbiosis negatively affects iron absorption, which in turn can lead to fatigue, mental "fog," depression, hair loss, restless leg syndrome, and even chronic heart disease. Research has even shown a direct correlation between the development of colon cancer and specific strains of harmful gut bacteria. In fact, a 2014 study published in the journal *Nature* has shown "unequivocal evidence" linking dysbiosis to the progression of a variety of cancers. A disturbing recent study shows that patients with cardiovascular disease, obesity, and type 2 diabetes often have dysbiosis, which promotes and accelerates their symptoms. Dysbiosis is also manifested in skin conditions such as eczema and dermatitis. And it can also cause bloating, constipation, or loose stools. It routinely rears its head as indigestion, heartburn, and GERD. You might assume that

THE WORD ON GERD (GASTROESOPHAGEAL REFLUX DISEASE) AND THE WILD MEDITERRANEAN DIET

GERD, or acid reflux, is the most costly gastrointestinal disease in the US, generating about $142 billion in direct and indirect costs. Yet few understand its underlying causes. Here's what happens: The esophagus and stomach are separated by a closure known as the lower esophageal sphincter (LES). When you've got a proper amount of acid in your stomach, the LES shuts to avoid having that acid damage the esophageal lining. When there's too little acid, however, the LES doesn't shut properly and some acidic fluid climbs back up into the esophagus. That's the burning sensation in GERD. There's another sphincter at the other end of the stomach that separates it from the small intestines. If the food in your stomach isn't properly digested, that door won't open. This leaves food sitting in your stomach to ferment, producing gas that leads to bloating and belching. So as you can see, what you don't want is low stomach acid!

This results in more than just discomfort. Your digestive system fails to break proteins into amino acids and bad bacteria can thrive in the microbiome. When acid levels are low, pathogens find a cozy atmosphere that allows them to overwhelm good bacteria.

Shifting to a Mediterranean diet high in plant fibers can definitely reduce symptoms of GERD. Some people also find relief in taking a daily dose of hydrochloric acid supplements, such as HCL and pepsin, at meal times to help increase the acid levels in the stomach. (You should not take HCL if you have stomach ulcers as it can be too harsh, and always consult your doctor before adding supplements to your diet.) Additionally, you can take a spoonful of apple cider vinegar in the mornings or eat a bit of raw cabbage daily, both of which have restorative impact on the gut. We'll talk more in Chapter 3 about how supplements, including HCL, can be used to increase stomach acid and combat the discomfort associated with GERD.

indigestion stems from excess stomach acid, but in truth, it's probably due to *low* stomach acid. Without enough digestive acids, your food isn't properly digested, causing it to be treated as a potentially dangerous invader and triggering an inflammatory response. What causes low stomach acid? Dysbiosis.

Dysbiosis occurs for a variety of reasons. The most common culprit is what we eat. Processed foods, an overdose of sugar, animal fats, hormone-laced dairy, fried foods, and artificially flavored or colored *anything* all have a negative impact on our guts, as do diets with too little plant-based fiber. Stress and being sedentary play a major role, too. Unnecessary use of antibiotics—and the CDC says about 30 percent of all antibiotic prescriptions fall into that category—can also throw the gut into disorder.

How Do I Know If My Gut Is Out of Whack?

The connection between how you feel and what might be happening in your gut isn't always apparent, which is why I order GI panels for *all* of my clients. In nine out of ten cases, my clients' results confirm a bacterial imbalance and buildup of pathogens. And sometimes we find the needle in the haystack that explains symptoms that have been baffling a client for a long time. I strongly recommend that you take one too. To learn more about the test I recommend, go to these websites for comprehensive stool tests/analyses:

www.doctorsdata.com

www.gdx.net

www.greatplainslaboratory.com

You can share this information with your healthcare provider if he or she isn't familiar with the test. You can also order a gut microbiome sequencing test from uBiome (ubiome.com).

Where Do We Go from Here?

By now it should be clear that the state of our digestive tracts has a powerful impact on our overall health.

And the foods we eat—plus the way we live (i.e., how much we move, how content we feel, how well we sleep)—can make the difference between a thriving digestive system and one that's sick. So our goal is to create a harmonious, healing state that balances the gut and restores wellness to the entire body.

Luckily, we can undo previous damage, whether it's been inflicted over a series of months or years. We can restore harmony to the gut and health to the body using concepts at the forefront of modern health advancement, which are—naturally—rooted in the sage wisdom of people who have been doing this for centuries. It's a process called "re-wilding," or reintroducing beneficial bacteria and microbes into the gut that have been either wiped out owing to things like overuse of antibiotics, or have been unable to flourish because of an overabundance of harmful pathogens. Think about it this way: Most of us live in a sterile world. We use antibacterial wipes to clean up, wash our hands with antibacterial soap, and eat irradiated or otherwise processed foods that lack from-the-soil nutrients and probiotic qualities that encourage beneficial bacterial growth. We also don't eat a broad

---

THE CONNECTION BETWEEN YOUR GUT AND YOUR THYROID

Between fifteen and twenty million Americans suffer from issues related to a malfunctioning thyroid. Most are plagued with hypothyroidism, a condition in which the thyroid produces too little hormone, resulting in a sluggish metabolism and a host of other symptoms including fatigue, dry skin, weight gain, depression, and mood swings. It's typically thought to be caused by damage from surgery or radiation, prescription medication, or lack of iodine in the diet, and the most widely accepted remedy is hormone replacement. So a patient is simply told to take pills for the rest of her life, and that's it.

However, researchers now believe there may be another cause: small intestine bacterial overgrowth, commonly known as SIBO.

SIBO is a chronic infection that occurs when bacteria that usually live in the GI tract experience an abnormal overgrowth and spill into the small intestine. While there are a variety of potential causes, excess sugar consumption is the most common.

If the hypothesis about SIBO being connected to thyroid health is correct, then it could spark a radical change in the treatment for hypothyroidism. Healing the bacteria overgrowth in the small intestine through diet and lifestyle could replace, or at least reduce, the need for hormone replacement in people suffering from thyroid issues.

enough *variety* of foods that are good for our gut. Our modern diet—which has become increasingly limited as fresh, plant-based foods and sustainably raised animal foods are less accessible than processed "convenience" foods—doesn't stoke the digestive system with the rich array of bacteria it's accustomed to (and needs in order to prevent disease). We consume only 10 percent as much fiber as our ancestors did on a daily basis. As a result, our guts aren't the wild places they need to be in order to thrive. Think about a fallow plot of land by the highway: The soil is packed and dry, most likely a little pale—not rich and black—and above all, has nothing growing in it but a few stray weeds. If you scooped up a handful, there'd be no bugs. Nothing can flourish in this environment, and you know why? Because it lacks the nutrients that support vital bacteria and microbes, which in turn encourage the growth of critters and plants. Your gut is no different. If we're going to get beautiful things growing again—to boost your energy; improve your sleep; maintain a healthy weight; clear up your skin; and alleviate chronic aches, pains, and illnesses—then we have work

> We can restore harmony to the gut and health to the body using concepts at the forefront of modern health advancement, which are—naturally—rooted in the sage wisdom of people who have been doing this for centuries.

to do. We need to remove detrimental bacteria and pathogens from the gut, flush your system with healing nutrients, and re-seed the gut with all the beneficial critters it needs. Plus, we need to get your body moving in a way that naturally boosts circulation and supports long-term homeostasis. Because your gut—and consequently your digestive system, immune system, neurological system, and just about every other element of your body—thrives on wild. It's what's called the 4 R's of creating harmony in your gut: Repair, Restore, Re-inoculate, and Rejuvenate.

And it all starts with a detox, or at least my version of it.

I developed this Wild Detox program to eliminate the foods that are disrupting the gut, while adding food-derived nutrients that will restore balance—specifically from Wild

Mediterranean foods and supplements that will help reintroduce beneficial flora to your microbiome. The first phase is the "pre-tox," during which we'll flood your body with plant fibers, the edible equivalent of a car detailing. This is followed by the "land-tox" or "sea-tox," customized detoxes that you'll read more about in the next chapter. I've come to believe that some people need the digestive boost that comes from the land's bounty (such as chicken, beef, root vegetables, and olive oil), foods that tend to be rich in conjugated linoleic acid (CLA) and omega-3s, which are powerful gut protectors and anti-inflammatories. Others require a jolt of minerals and proteins that come from the sea (such as those found in fish and sea vegetables). These foods are loaded with zinc, vitamin D, and magnesium, which aid mucosal healing, normalize glucose levels via the gut, and improve mood and reduce anxiety, respectively. Fish and sea vegetables also aid the absorption of iodine in the small intestine, making them excellent for thyroid health. As opposed to nutrition's traditionally one-size-fits-all approach, this method allows you to choose what suits your unique physiological disposition best—something I'll help you determine with a quiz on page 67. This detox process is a crucial first step toward recreating harmony in your gut and balancing your system, and also acquainting you with what it means to have a "wild kitchen," one that harnesses the power of eating a diversity of Mediterranean foods. These are foods that have proven for hundreds of years to support our bodies in ways "experts" only just now realize can help alleviate many of our health problems, both because they pack a hefty nutritional punch and also because they offer the opportunity to eat a diverse diet—a crucial element for stocking your gut with a wide range of beneficial, health-boosting bacteria.

> I've come to believe that some people need the digestive boost that comes from the land's bounty. Others require a jolt of minerals and proteins that come from the sea.

I've dedicated this program to helping you make that happen. Unlike fad diets and fancy meal plans, the lifestyle based on living wild and the foods of the Mediterranean is time-tested. It has enabled people to thrive for hundreds of years. I've just updated it by combining ancient wisdom with modern science.

Fat vs. Lean Microbes

You may have been drawn to this book in part because you're interested in losing weight. Everyone knows that obesity is a major problem not just in the United States, but in many countries throughout the world. Unfortunately, people of every age, gender, class, and ethnicity struggle with their weight.

But I'm going to suggest switching your goal from losing weight to making digestive health your number-one priority. That's why I don't provide a caloric menu for my program. Too often, people associate foods primarily with the calories they contain, not with their other nutritional values. (Artificial sweeteners are a great example. They're low-calorie, but researchers have discovered that they—specifically aspartame and saccharin—can alter gut bacteria in a way that causes our blood sugar levels to spike, leading to type 2 diabetes and heart disease.) It's also worth mentioning that certain additives—such as processed sugar, saturated fats, and MSG—trigger us to crave those very items. When we get a hit of sweet/artificially savory/greasy, we are wired to want more. It's our brain's dirty little trick for getting us to eat foods that pack the biggest caloric punch. But we don't need to scavenge for our food anymore. (And we certainly don't need to eat foods that have been chemically engineered to taste good, either.) Instead, I want you to think of the food you take in as the way you nourish yourself and strengthen your health via your microbiome. Once you experience the amazing power of gut balance through food and lifestyle choices and your body begins to absorb the crucial micronutrients needed for full-throttle metabolism, you'll find that you will feel a lot less discomfort *and* lose weight in the bargain.

In fact, scientists are now discovering that gut bacteria are powerful players in whether or not you hold on to fat. A 2014 study conducted by researchers from Cornell University and King's College, London, compared intestinal bacteria in obese and lean individuals. The study concluded that the gut ecosystems in thin people flourish with a wide variety of bacteria, specifically the kind that can break down starches and fibers into shorter molecules, which the body then uses as energy. On the other hand, the study showed that the gut environment in heavier people is imbalanced and much less diverse. (I suspect this is partly due to a lower intake of plant fibers on the part of the overweight individuals—something we'll get to later.) An imbalance in gut flora can negatively affect your metabolism. If your levels of a beneficial bacteria fall too low, it can lead to decreased levels of TSH, a crucial hormone that impacts your thyroid and slows your metabolism, making it difficult to lose weight.

This leads me to a couple of mice I'd like to introduce you to. That big guy? He's Big Jim. That lean little fella? He's Mini Fred. In a study led by a Harvard researcher, obese mice like Big Jim were injected with a fecal implant from a lean mouse like Mini Fred. The idea was that such an implant would change the profile of the bacteria in the intestines of the obese mice. The result? The fat mice experienced rapid weight loss. While we don't know for certain if such methods would work in humans, the bottom line is clear: A healthy, balanced gut is good for the waistline.

My Promise to You

You might think your health issues are unavoidable, whether it's struggling with digestive discomfort, extra weight, low energy, headaches, skin problems, or other health maladies. Maybe some of these issues run in your family. But your genes are not your entire destiny. We now know that our microbiota can actually influence epigenetic factors, or gene expressions that are passed down from generation to generation and woven into our DNA. Factors like body weight, physical activity, dietary fac-

> Change your gut, and you can change your life.

tors, and environmental toxins can all affect—and be affected by—the gut microbiome. So it stands to reason—and has been proven in studies—that if you change your weight, physical activity, dietary factors, and exposure to environmental toxins, you no longer need to fall prey to conditions once thought to be a life sentence. Change your gut, and you can change your life. So let's get you started on reconnecting to your gut, your wild side, and your true health.

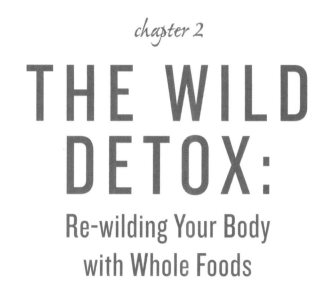

chapter 2

THE WILD DETOX:

Re-wilding Your Body
with Whole Foods

> "When you get close to the raw materials and taste them at the moment they let go of the soil, you learn to respect them."
>
> René Redzepi, chef/owner, Noma

SEARCH THE INTERNET FOR THE WORD "DETOX" AND YOU'LL GET OVER 100 MILLION HITS, WITH programs based on everything from raw food, green juice, soups, teas, herbs, lemon water, and eliminating sugar, to cabbage, protein shakes, cranberry juice, and even eggs. Detox is big business, a booming part of the $60 billion diet industry.

Perhaps you have tried some kind of detox before. After all, they're often touted as the magic solution to all that ails us. And the diet industry is complicit. Detox products have seen massive growth in the marketplace, in part because many of them *seem* to work. Usually this has less to do with the regimen or product itself than it does with what you *remove* from your diet during the cleanse—namely processed foods, high-fructose corn syrup and other processed sugars, alcohol, and caffeine. But, because there's typically no plan for reentering the real world of food and living day-to-day life, when the detox ends, slowly but surely the old symptoms started to creep back.

It's for all these reasons that I'm hesitant to even use the word "detox." The process that I believe is key to restoring your well-being isn't an extreme diet or a short-term solution to a long-term problem. After all, you wouldn't expect that fallow plot of land I mentioned earlier to suddenly burst into bloom overnight, right? And your well-being is certainly not nurtured by a bunch of expensive potions. Rather, consider this simple but powerful approach: Use real food. Full stop. The old saying that "you are what you eat" is strikingly true when it comes to your digestive system. Just *one* meal can rapidly sway the state of your gut, pendulum-style.

Using the nutrients and fibers that naturally reside in real, whole foods you can start to reboot your system. As hundreds of my clients have found, following this plan, then shifting to a Wild Mediterranean diet will help keep your gut balanced for the long haul.

The Wild Detox Playbook

Consider me your detox coach. Like all coaches, I've developed a playbook, or set of rules and strategies, to help my clients understand what I'm prescribing and why.

In general, the Wild Detox is composed of two parts: a "pre-tox" and then either a "land-tox" or a "sea-tox." The pre-tox is like a deep cleaning for your gut. It's a three-day period during which you're giving your body a rest from immunogenic foods—those foods that could be giving your immune system a hard time, including processed foods, soy, dairy, wheat, eggs, and corn—while simultaneously flooding your system with tons of Mediterranean diet–specific plants, plus some lean proteins and healthy fats. Why? Because plants—i.e., fruits and vegetables—are the ultimate gut healers. And unlike a commercial juice cleanse, where plants are reduced to their sugary, fiberless components, eating whole plants sends things like polysaccharides, lipids, and peptides through your digestive system to create the best environment for growing rich gut microbiota. While they're busy recolonizing beneficial bacteria and balancing the gut, they also bind to harmful pathogens and bacteria and escort them out of the body. This puts the body in perfect position to start receiving all the nutrients that we're flooding it with—including all the protein, lipids, vitamins, and minerals that lean proteins and healthy fats provide. It's a whole-food approach that demonstrates just how curative food, and in particular the ingredients of the Mediterranean, can be.

The next phase of the Wild Detox is either a land-tox or sea-tox. After taking the quiz on page 67 to determine which is a better fit for you, you'll spend the following three days eating Wild Mediterranean foods that have particularly curative powers for your specific needs. On a sea-tox, foods such as seafood and seaweed give your body a burst of minerals like iodine and fatty acids such as DHA. The lean meats, fats, and plants of a land-tox pack a diversity of healthy fatty acids and plant fiber, a potent combination that aids in the uptake of micronutrients. While these detoxes are especially formulated to suit various conditions, please note that your body would be happy to have either!

The foods you'll eat during this three-day period are crucial for rewiring your addictions to processed sugars and fats as well as rebuilding gut health, but there's another extremely important element that I'll be adding: intermittent fasting. We'll talk much more about this later in the chapter, but rest assured, it's not as scary as it sounds. You won't go hungry, and it's one of the best things you can do for your body as it heals and re-wilds.

The last phase of the Wild Detox is transitioning back to a style of eating that's not so much a diet as it is a lifelong mind-set. At this point you will have seen just how incredible you

PRE-DETOX SELF-TEST

1. Do you have constant food cravings?
   (Y) (N)

2. Gas and bloating (Y) (N)

3. Immune system
   (A) You have flu-like symptoms more than 3 times per year.
   (B) Sick 2 to 3 times per year.
   (C) Rarely get sick.

4. Sleeping habits
   (A) You get less than 5 hours of sleep per night.
   (B) Sleep 5 to 6 hours per night.
   (C) Sleep 7 to 8 hours of uninterrupted sleep per night.

5. Mental fog: You have a decreased ability to focus, lack of clear thinking, and memory loss. (Y) (N)

6. Fatigue and energy crashes: Do you have difficulties waking in the morning or hit slumps throughout the day? (Y) (N)

7. Skin breakouts or rashes? (Y) (N)

8. Digestion
   (A) Often constipated
   (B) Eliminate 1 time per day
   (C) Eliminate 2 to 3 times per day

Scores:
If you answered yes to any of the Y/N questions, add 3 points.
For the other questions:
(A) = 3 points
(B) = 2 points
(C) = 0

Results:
0–3 = You're pretty healthy but should consider a pre-tox at least once a year for maintenance.

3–15 = A pre-tox right now is going to benefit you tremendously. I also recommend a pre-tox every 3 months, followed by a lard-tox or sea-tox.

15+ = I recommend a regular pre-tox program, completing one every 6 weeks, followed by a land-tox or sea-tox every 3 months.

can feel when all of your body's systems are working the way they should. To help you resist the temptation to go back to your old eating habits, I'll show you instead how to add foods back into the rotation in a way that's mindful. If, say, resuming your morning protein shakes leaves you feeling sluggish and bloated, then you may be reacting to some of the artificial ingredients found in commercial protein powders, and that's your body's way of saying that it's not such a big fan of that particular item. The same goes for all the foods we initially took away (soy, dairy, eggs, wheat, corn). The goal isn't to eventually reinstate all the foods you used to eat, as that's most likely how you wound up feeling not so great in the first place. Rather you'll learn what works for you and say good-bye—perhaps permanently—to what doesn't. In the next chapter, we'll explore all the delicious options that exist in a Wild Mediterranean diet and talk about how to incorporate all these foods into your diet. And to help you see how many (extremely delicious) gut-balancing options you have—which is important because eating a diversity of foods is just as important as opting for healthier ones—I've dedicated an entire section of "village-to-table" recipes starting on page 92. The "village-to-table" approach I advocate takes advantage of the foods and cooking methods used for generations in countries like Greece, Spain, France, and Italy—which have been the foundation for health in those communities.

Getting Started: Preparing to Detox

Unlike other detox programs that require at least a week of scaling back the foods you eat, I want you to immediately stop eating foods that could be irritating your gut, cold turkey, and start giving your body a gentle scrub with lots and lots of plant fibers—specifically, a 3:1 ratio of veggies to lean proteins. To help you have the most success, I recommend these simple preparations:

- **CLEAR YOUR SCHEDULE.** It's best if you commit to this process 100 percent, which is why I developed a program that is 6 days long, shorter than most other detoxes. Because it's not 14 or 30 days long, you'll need to accomplish more in less time. That means that you have to give it your all. That means 6 total days where you aren't interrupting the detox and introducing other foods. This allows the gut to heal and means you won't be upsetting your digestive system when it's vulnerable. Have a wedding to go to this week-end and know you'll be too tempted by those passed appetizers? Going on a road trip? Hold off, and start your pre-tox the next week.

• **CLEAN OUT YOUR KITCHEN**. This is the time when you finally say good-bye to foods that aren't doing your system any favors. I mean it; get rid of them. It's not worth the temptation, and besides, you'll need to make room for all the incredible, healing foods we'll talk about later in this chapter. Here's what you'll need to toss:

The Foul Five

These are foods that have no place in your life, whether you're detoxing or not. They contain ingredients that actively upset the balance in your digestive system such as processed sugar; artificial flavoring, coloring, or sweetening; additives; texturizers; preservatives; and other nasty elements that are causing full-body problems. Even that yogurt that claims to be "all-natural" or the crackers labeled "GMO-free"—ditch 'em. Most packaged and processed foods, even those sold in health food stores, contain some preservatives, sweeteners, or other additives.

I. CURED AND PROCESSED MEATS (think bologna, sausages, bacon, and ham)

2. PROCESSED SUGAR AND ARTIFICIAL SWEETENERS, including any food that lists sugar, corn sugar, high-fructose corn syrup, aspartame, maltitol, sorbitol, etc. as an ingredient

3. REFINED GRAIN PRODUCTS (white flour, de-germed cornmeal, white bread, crackers, breads, most breakfast cereals, some pastas—basically any item that doesn't come from a whole grain)

4. PROCESSED SOY can be found in things like soybean oil, yogurt, protein powders, chips, and energy bars. (On the other hand, unprocessed organic soy, like tempeh, miso, and edamame can be healthy additions to your diet.)

5. FRIED FOODS (enough said)

The Finicky Five

While these aren't necessarily "bad" foods, they can be immunogenic or trigger an inflammatory response in people whose guts are out of balance. Because there's currently no test on the market that can reliably indicate whether you have a food intolerance, the only way to be sure is to first eliminate suspected immunogenic foods, and then re-introduce them one at a time. That's why I recommend avoiding them during Wild Detox, so that you can be certain that nothing is irritating your digestive system. By adding them back in gradually, you'll be able to identify symptoms that indicate whether this food might not be a good fit for you. It may not always be on the "no" list, though; as your gut continues to heal, you might develop the ability to eat these foods once again.

1. EGGS
2. UNPROCESSED ORGANIC SOY
3. DAIRY
4. GLUTEN
5. CORN

Let me tell you about my client Grady, a professional Ironman triathlete. His experience is a great example of the power of the pre-tox. He came to see me while in the off-season when he wasn't in training. Grady was suffering from chronic respiratory infections, which isn't uncommon with elite athletes. Each morning, he would train hard and then hit a major slump around 1 p.m. A lot of my clients report afternoon doldrums when they first come to see me, but mostly that complaint comes from women. Usually, men report trouble falling asleep. Grady checked his blood sugar and discovered that it would dip very low, to around 55 mg/dl, in the afternoon.

First we removed everything in his current diet regimen. I'm talking about a total overhaul. Right away, he suffered from flu-like symptoms, including all-over body aches. He called to tell me he was unable to get out of bed. I asked him to try and stick with it for seventy-two hours. He did. By the end of the second day, he was feeling much better. By day three, he felt very different. His stools had improved dramatically. By day four, he called to tell me that he felt as if he was floating on Cloud Nine.

Many clients prefer to stay on the pre-tox for some time. They like the structure, plus the foods are bland so when they change up and cook for themselves or go out to eat, the food nearly explodes with flavor, another interesting way to retrain your palate.

During the pre-tox, Grady had one very telling experience when he attended a sporting industry function and ate some conventional (most likely laden with corn syrup or processed sugar) granola bars provided by the event's sponsors. His newly balanced gut didn't care for them at all; he said it felt as if he were carrying bricks in his stomach.

Now Grady feeds his elite-athlete body with a plant-rich, wild protein, and fat-approved Mediterranean diet. He replaced his highly processed, artificially colored, sugar-infused protein powders with a version that is made from dehydrated grass-fed beef.

• **STOCK YOUR DETOX PANTRY.** Buy enough veggies, lean proteins, and healthy fats to get you through the next six days. While we'll talk more about the specific health benefits of each of these foods later in the chapter, for now, take this list to the grocery store and consider these items your new best friends:

- ☐ Fish (cod, sardines, salmon, halibut, sole, scallops, shrimp)
- ☐ Organic chicken or turkey (fresh or frozen)
- ☐ Organic frozen berries (any kind), the only approved fruit
- ☐ Broccoli
- ☐ Cucumbers
- ☐ Celery
- ☐ Carrots
- ☐ Cabbage
- ☐ Garlic
- ☐ Jerusalem artichokes (sunchokes)
- ☐ Organic mushrooms
- ☐ Lettuce, any kind
- ☐ Onions
- ☐ Fresh or dried herbs such as rosemary, parsley, oregano, thyme, and sage
- ☐ Lemons
- ☐ Sweet potatoes
- ☐ Brown rice
- ☐ Sauerkraut
- ☐ Dried seaweed sheets (nori)
- ☐ Extra-virgin olive oil
- ☐ Coconut oil

• **INVEST IN A FEW KEY SUPPLEMENTS.** I know I told you that you didn't need to buy fancy potions for the Wild Detox, but these are in no way similar to the dubious "cure-alls" that companies sell with the promise that you'll lose 20 pounds in 10 days. These supplements are intended to support all the body's systems while helping to reverse damage, promote healing, and fill in all the nutritional "blanks" left by an unbalanced diet. Plus, nobody's perfect. There're always going to be the demands of everyday life, and when they creep in, sometimes even the best of intentions can go out the window. Or consider that, when it comes to the gut, "stress" isn't just caused by things like being stuck in traffic or getting in an argument. Stress can also mean sitting in a desk chair all day long (not giving the gut enough circulation), or even watching something inadvertently stressful on TV. These supplements—particularly the adaptogens, in the case of better handling stress— are like having a little healthy safety net. They can all be found in a health food store or online, with the exception of the topical mineral spray, which you can make at home with a few simple ingredients (see page 202). Here are the others I recommend. You can find my favorite brands in the Resources section on page 209.

- **Adaptogens:** Adaptogens are a family of herbs that I could never live without. They are truly Mother Nature's gift for the adrenal glands. I have tested the placebo effect with adaptogens, and it's clear that they are, indeed, delivering powerful benefits. They give a boost of *sustained* energy throughout the day (no caffeine required) because they help keep blood sugar stable. They help regulate the appetite, aid in post-workout recovery, and calm the nervous system (a lifesaver for anyone dealing with stress—and who isn't?—or anxiety). Adaptogens can boost mental and physical performance, as well as longevity. Because they're so beneficial to the circulatory system, they're also a boon for anyone struggling with erectile dysfunction. And as if that weren't enough, they have also been found to have an antidiabetic effect. My top picks are Siberian ginseng, ashwagandha, gotu kola, and licorice root. Pick one and, if you like it, slowly add more to your rotation.

- **Food-based multivitamin:** I always recommend an organic food-based multivitamin over synthetic. For one thing, it doesn't exactly seem "healthy" when your urine is stained bright orange from lab-made carotenoids, or carries a distinct vitamin smell. Plus, research suggests that synthetic vitamins can actually be detrimental to your health. Folate is a group of water-soluble B vitamins (the synthetic form is folic acid) that has been linked to an increased risk of autistic children when taken by pregnant women, and synthetic B_6 and B_{12} have been linked to an increase in cancers. As for vitamin D—the crucial vitamin responsible for healthy bones and teeth, circulation, and defense from myriad diseases—I don't love getting it from a vitamin at all, namely because there's inconclusive long-term research about how much supplemental vitamin D is too much (because it can be toxic), or if it's even a sufficient substitute. I recommend getting your daily dose from foods rich in vitamin D, such as fatty fish and egg yolks, as well as exposure to early-morning and late-afternoon sunlight. After all, people living in the Mediterranean have lived long, healthy lives without supplementing!

PROBIOTIC SUPPLEMENTS

It's reasonable to assume that if we're talking about re-wilding your gut, or reseeding it with lots of beneficial bacteria, that I'd recommend taking a probiotic supplement. After all, probiotics have become all the rage in food marketing, from yogurt products to kombucha. While that's certainly the right idea, unfortunately you can't rely on a pill to give your gut the balanced diversity of bacteria it needs. Most supplements contain less than seven strains of bacteria, when 300 to 500 bacterial strains, which include more than 2 million genes, exist in an optimally stocked gut.

That's what makes eating a diversity of whole, wild foods the better solution for getting all the probiotic power your digestive system needs in order to thrive. And I'm not just talking about yogurt, the usual probiotic go-to. In fact, yogurt isn't the perfect food that we—or food marketers—have made it out to be. Like most processed dairy products you'll find in the grocery store, yogurt has been pasteurized or heated to kill off any potential damaging bacteria, taking all the good stuff with it, too. Manufacturers will add certain strains of bacteria back in, but the nutritional integrity has already been compromised. A much better option is including probiotic-rich fermented foods (page 59) in your diet, and at least eight servings of vegetables—all that plant fiber is ideal for flora building!

If you're relying on a supplement to get all the good stuff—instead of getting them from whole, "wild" foods, as this program recommends—then you're not only limiting the probiotic diversity of your gut, but you also risk getting too much of a good thing. That's right: Overdoing it on probiotic supplements or processed products (including kombucha, which is fermented) can lead to a detrimental overload. The key is to create balance with the foods you're eating.

- Bee pollen/royal jelly: These food sources for bees and their colonies are nature's elixirs. They help balance the hormones and ease PMS symptoms, promote oral health, strengthen the immune system, and most notably, have anti-inflammatory and antioxidant properties in the GI tract, making them perfect supplements for supporting gut health.

- Prebiotics: Prebiotic fibers are an important part of gut health, if not *the* most important—perhaps more so even than probiotic-rich foods. Prebiotic fibers are nondigestible, meaning they sail through our GI tract without being broken down. And when they arrive at our gut, they're eagerly gobbled up by the beneficial critters who live there. They're also important for your metabolism because they enhance how the body can absorb and use macronutrients like carbohydrates and protein, as well as minerals. Boosting your prebiotic intake is also associated with having an easier time shedding extra weight. There are certain foods that have prebiotic benefits—which I'll talk more about on page 60—but I still recommend taking a supplement, especially during the detox process. To source your supplement, look for reputable brands who sell inulin, a type of prebiotic fiber.

- Spirulina: Spirulina is a bright-green algae that has a long list of nutritional benefits. It's high in protein, bioavailable iron, and B vitamins; and it's loaded with antioxidants. You can take it either in tablet or powder form.

- Topical mineral spray: If you don't have access to clean sea or ocean water, I recommend making the Wild Mediterranean Sea Spray (page 202). Sea salt is packed with minerals, can boost circulation, has anti-inflammatory properties, and has been shown to mitigate the effects of coronary heart disease. I would often accompany my grandmother to the therapeutic sea water baths of Methana, Greece, where soaking in sea water is an age-old remedy known for its restorative powers.

- Powdered protein: No, not like the creatine the guys at the gym are pounding, rather clean, food-derived sources of protein that can easily be mixed into a shake for a gentle boost of energy. I don't recommend whey protein (isolate or concentrate), because most of my clients report that it leaves them feeling bloated and unsatisfied. If you eat meat, then my top choice is Designs for Health HydroBEEF (www.designsforhealth.com). This supplement gives you the same benefits of animal proteins—namely loads of energy because the amino acids are metabolized into energy by glucose and fatty acids, without the headaches or crash you feel after taking a synthetic energizing supplement. I also like high-quality goat-based protein powder (Garden of Life or Meyenberg), though it may be difficult to tolerate if you have dairy sensitivity. If you're vegetarian/vegan, look for pea or brown rice proteins that are bonded with other nutrients, such as organic grasses: Amazing Grass (www.amazinggrass.com) and Vega One (myvega.com). I have found that these work for my clients who tell me that powders that are less nutrient-rich leave them feeling hungry.

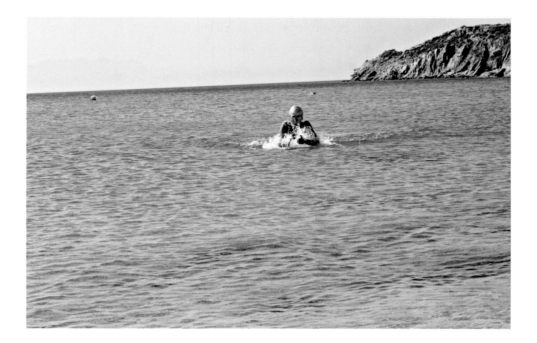

DO I HAVE TO GIVE UP CAFFEINE?

The first time I put my mother on a detox, I casually mentioned that cutting coffee was part of the process. She gave me one of those, "I'm-the-mother-you're-the-child-don't-be-telling-me-what-to-do" kind of looks. So I know what you're thinking when I say that you need to make do without the caffeine. Don't worry! It's not forever.

However, as part of the detoxing process, I always ask people to cut out caffeine as much as possible since it can cause erratic insulin levels in some people. If you're a diehard morning coffee drinker like my mother, I recommend mixing half a cup of coffee with hot water so you get the same warm moment in the morning while still cutting back caffeine. An added bonus comes if you stir in some fat—such as coconut oil or even butter—which helps minimize the sugar spike caused by fluctuating glucose levels.

When you add caffeine back into your daily routine, I recommend that you be on the lookout for symptoms that it may be affecting you in an adverse way. For starters, check your blood sugar before and after drinking a caffeinated beverage to make sure that you are not experiencing spikes in your blood sugar levels. (Simply follow the manufacturer's instructions or go to WebMD to watch the video on checking your blood sugar: www.webmd.com/diabetes/video/how-to-check-your-blood-sugar.) Even without testing your blood, you might be able tell if your insulin levels increase noticeably if you find yourself hungry after drinking that cup of coffee or tea.

Second, does caffeine make you feel bloated or cause any type of gastrointestinal distress? This could be a sign that caffeine may be altering your gut—and not in a good way.

If you experience any of these side effects, try giving up coffee for a week, which could help to develop a more stable environment in your biome. If you struggle with cravings for coffee, try putting a small amount in hot water as I suggested above, or cut your intake to a half cup.

I'm no stranger to caffeine dependence. There was a time when I relied on coffee to get me through the day. I found myself craving sugary foods, a result of the irregularities in my blood sugar. I finally had to admit that my gut simply couldn't handle a daily coffee habit. Now, I indulge in coffee as a special treat when I get together with friends. On most days, though, I sip unsmoked yerba maté—a drink made from a plant whose leaves have the power of coffee but the healing benefits of tea. Indigenous peoples have used it for centuries as a social and medicinal beverage, and modern research shows it could protect DNA from oxidation and has a high antioxidant capacity.

Invest in Tests

In my practice, I recommend a number of diagnostic tests for clients, which help us get a clear picture of what's going on in their unique systems. Because it's difficult for you to administer these tests and then interpret the results without a trained professional, I suggest simply sticking with two extremely easy at-home tests: blood sugar monitoring and the hydrochloric acid tests. However, I've also included the full list of tests I like to run, in the event that your health-care professional offers these screenings.

At-Home Tests

Blood Sugar Monitor

You may think that blood sugar testing is just for individuals dealing with diabetes. On the contrary, a glucose monitor (which you can buy at the drugstore or online) can give insight into which foods might be spiking your blood sugar and, in turn, negatively affecting the balance of your microbiota. Blood sugar testing also offers an inexpensive way to understand the underlying reason you might feel exhausted by midafternoon or you have difficulty sleeping at night. By harnessing the power of blood sugar testing, you'll discover how your body responds to various foods and lifestyle habits.

As you now know, everyone's microbiome and metabolic system is as unique as a fingerprint. In my case, I was surprised to discover that eating a lot of white rice and the amount of coffee I was drinking led to my own blood sugar irregularities, which means that I now try to omit (or at least limit) these foods to protect the balance in my gut and generally feel better.

To see more specifically what might be affecting your blood sugar, I recommend purchasing a monitor and then using it a couple days before your pre-tox (during your "normal" routine) and then during your pre-tox, testing right after you wake up and then again after each meal. That said, I realize that it might not be the easiest thing to do at work, in which case, you can still get accurate results if you limit testing to first thing in the morning and after larger meals. Track your results by writing them down or inputting them into an app such as Glucose Buddy or OnTrack Diabetes. You're looking for irregularities, particularly any foods that prompt your blood sugar level to rise above 130 mg/dl or dip below 70 mg/dl. Because you'll be eating simple meals made up of just a few components (more on this in a bit), it should be fairly easy to identify the culprit. Consider removing that food from your diet moving forward.

A blood sugar monitor also comes in handy for identifying when your blood sugar may be too low. Many of my clients report waking in the night, which can be the result of blood sugar irregularities. If this is a problem for you, the next time you find yourself up at the wee hours of the night, test your blood sugar. If it's low (below 70 mg/dl), take a bite of wild-approved protein (pages 56 to 57) along with some fat, such as a bit of olive oil, to help even out your levels.

Hydrochloric Acid Test

As I mentioned in Chapter 2, many common digestive problems, including GERD and small intestinal bacterial overgrowth, are the result of *low* stomach acid. If you have any digestive issues at all, one of the first things you need to do is determine whether or not you have low stomach acid. There are a couple ways to do this, but the most reliable at-home method is the Betaine HCL challenge test. Don't fall for expensive online "kits" for this.

1. Purchase 650 mg Betaine HCL supplements with pepsin.
2. Take one 650 mg capsule 15 minutes before eating.
3. Eat at least 6 ounces of wild-approved protein (pages 56 to 57). (This is important as too little protein can yield a false positive.)
4. Halfway through your meal, take another pill.
5. Finish eating your meal, paying attention to how your body reacts.

Important Note Nonsteroidal anti-inflammatory drugs (NSAIDs) and corticosteroids increase the chances of ulcers in the stomach and together with Betaine HCL increase the risk of gastritis. Consult a physician before trying this test or supplementing.

There are two possible outcomes from this test: You might not notice any difference, which indicates that you likely have low stomach acid. Or you may experience a sense of heaviness, burning, or "heat" in your abdomen, which signals that you do not have low acid levels. A glass of water mixed with ½ teaspoon baking soda will relieve the discomfort. A less precise but less scary version of this test can be performed with simple baking soda. Mix ¼ teaspoon baking soda in 8 ounces cold water and consume first thing in the morning, before eating or drinking anything except water. The baking soda will react with the acid in your stomach to create carbon dioxide gas, which in turn should cause you to burp up that gas. Time how long it takes to belch. If your stomach is producing adequate amounts of hydrochloric acid you should probably belch within 2 to 3 minutes. Early and repeated belching may be due to excessive stomach acid. If you have not belched within 5 minutes you have low acid levels in your stomach.

I recommend doing this test a couple of times throughout your pre-tox to confirm your reaction. If you have two positive results, then it's time to start regularly supplementing with Betaine HCL to increase your stomach acid levels and improve your digestive functions. Start with two or three capsules a day, then gradually reduce the number of capsules needed, perhaps only taking one if you're having a protein-heavy meal. As noted on the previous page, be sure to discuss with your physician before adding HCL to your diet.

Ask Your Doctor

This full workup can provide insight into everything from underlying inflammation and hormone imbalance to the presence of viruses and thyroid dysfunction.

- **GI panel** (including a comprehensive stool analysis)
- **Microbiology profile**
- **Life Extension weight-loss panel** (basic and comprehensive)
- **Full blood panel,** including sex hormones (DHEA-S, free and total testosterone, estradiol [E2], and progesterone), thyroid hormones (TSH, free T3, free T4, and reverse T3), stress hormones (cortisol), insulin resistance markers (insulin, ferritin, hemoglobin A1C), inflammation and general health markers (complete metabolic panel, lipid panel, CBC, vitamin D 25-hydroxy, and C-reactive protein)
- **Urinalysis**

Best Ingredients for Your Detox

During your pre-tox your food choices will be governed by one simple rule of thumb: Eat only foods that consist of a single ingredient. That ensures that the meals you create will be made of foods that have no additives, no flavorings, no artificial coloring—nothing besides what nature gave them. Carrots. Broccoli. Chicken breast. Salmon. Olive oil. Sea salt. The beauty of these foods is that they don't contain the antigens that set off the TLR receptors I mentioned in Chapter 1, causing an unnecessary attack that saps the body of resources and causes inflammation. Let's take a closer look at the list of foods to stock up on that I shared earlier in the chapter, so you understand *why* I want you to have them handy.

> **Key Foods and How to Prepare Them for This Program:**
>
> **P** = Pre-tox friendly
> **L** = Land-tox friendly
> **S** = Sea-tox friendly

LETTUCES, OF ALL VARIETIES P L are, first and foremost, rich in fiber. This is critical for positively influencing the metabolic activity of the microbiome, specifically by contributing to the number of short-chain fatty acids (SCFA), which are super important for intestinal health, especially because they're the main source of energy for the cells in your colon.

They're also high in vitamin K, which boosts energy and metabolism while quelling inflammation; as well as heart-healthy B vitamin folate; the blood-building nutrient iron; fiber; vitamin C; potassium, and plant-based omega-3 fatty acids. And they're high in mineral-rich water content and packed with phytonutrients. Use lettuces as a base for a salad dressed with Wild Vinaigrette (page 173), a drizzle of olive oil, or even a mix of equal-parts butter and olive oil (1 tablespoon each). That's right—fat is your friend when it comes to salads (in fact, all veggies), because fats (unlike reduced-fat or fat-free dressings) help the body absorb the plants' nutrients. Lettuces are subject to intense pesticide spraying, so be sure to purchase organic.

CABBAGE P L S The humble cabbage is part of a class of vegetables called the cruciferous family known for its sulfur-containing, cancer-preventive substances such as indole-3-

carbinol. Cabbage, in particular, contains sulforaphane, which helps stimulate the production of detoxifying enzymes in the metabolsim, making cabbage a natural detox companion. And all the flavonoids that come with cabbage's polyphenolic compounds are incredibly beneficial for GI tract health, and in turn, gut health. I advise consuming cabbage at least two or three times per week. For the detox, cabbage may be shredded and combined with romaine as a base for salad or steamed and eaten with a power protein, such as braised meats, steamed fish, or roasted poultry.

SWEET POTATOES 🅿 🇱 These are the best starch-based carbohydrates you can buy, because, first, those polysaccharides (carbohydrates that provide energy storage or structural support) are potent prebiotics, a digestive stimulant that's crucial for the gut re-wilding that we'll talk about in more detail later in the chapter. Sweet potatoes also contain vitamin B_6, which helps with protein digestion in the gut. Their golden orange color comes from the naturally occurring beta-carotene, a potent antioxidant for overall health benefits. I always recommend having sweet potatoes on hand—they're so rich in vitamins, minerals, and fiber, and incredibly versatile. Simply boil them, or bake them, either seasoned with salt or tossed with herbs or spices.

BERRIES 🅿 🇱 No diet should be without these powerful antioxidant and pigment-rich super fruits! Their inflammation-fighting compounds work their magic bodywide, including in the gut, which helps maintain a healthy balance of microbiota. From their cardio-protective and neurological health benefits (thanks, vitamin C!), to blood sugar stabilization, berries are considered a powerhouse of nutrients. Preferred types of berries are strawberries, raspberries, blueberries, blackberries, and red and black currants. Both fresh and frozen berries are superior sources of antioxidants. Like lettuces, conventional berries are drenched in pesticides, so opt for organic.

OLIVE OIL 🅿 🇱 You should have a quality extra-virgin olive oil in your kitchen at all times. It's a major part of the Mediterranean diet, and it so happens that a diet rich in extra-virgin olive oil can increase certain strains of beneficial bacteria in the gut, namely bifidobacteria, which have been associated with alleviating gastrointestinal disorders such as inflammatory bowel disease. Researchers have found that olive oil in the diet is linked to increased intestinal immunity, decreased inflammation, and overall wellness of the digestive system. When eaten raw and paired with plant fiber, olive oil can help increase the number of beneficial flora in your gut—and the more diverse and balanced the good guys are, the more robust your immune system will be.

Olive oil is also rich in phenolic compounds, which have anti-inflammatory, antimicrobial, antibacterial, and antiviral properties. Plus it's loaded with monounsaturated fat (which has been linked to a decreased risk for breast cancer, reduced cholesterol levels, lower risk for heart disease and stroke, weight loss, and relief from arthritis-related discomfort) and a long list of phytonutrients. Use this as your main fat, whether for cooking or drizzling on salads.

NUTS AND SEEDS 🅿 🅛 Humans have been eating nuts and seeds for millennia. They remain one of the healthiest snack foods available, especially if you choose raw, unsalted over roasted or seasoned varieties. They contain natural fibers and phytochemicals that help facilitate the presence of healthy and diverse bacteria. And like olive oil, they're full of antiviral, bioavailable selenium (meaning your body can easily access and absorb it), magnesium, and monounsaturated fat. Because they contain vitamin E with mixed tocopherols and tocotrienols, they are considered the "king" of antioxidants, magnesium, and monounsaturated fat. They're a terrific addition to salads and make handy snacks when you're on the go.

ROAST TURKEY 🅿 🅛 In addition to protein, selenium, tryptophan, vitamins B_3 and B_6, and phosphorus, roast turkey contains zinc, which is commonly deficient in most people and aids mucosal healing (crucial for the kind of work we're doing with this detox because mucosal surfaces in our body—such as the gut—have a big impact on immune system and metabolic function). I recommend cooking your own at home instead of purchasing deli turkey, which is typically processed with nitrates and sodium. Roast a whole or half breast and you'll never go a week without having this beneficial protein in your refrigerator. A simple way to prepare it is to slather the breast with olive oil, sprinkle it with a bit of salt, and season with dried herbs such as thyme, sage, and rosemary. Roast at 375°F for about 15 minutes per pound, or until an instant-read thermometer registers 165°F. Select organic turkey when you can.

GRASS-FED BEEF 🄿 🄻 Beef is rich in gut-friendly nutrients like zinc as well as B_{12}, which is now thought to be a major contributor to helping beneficial microbes flourish. Eating foods rich in B_{12} is a little like helping your gut microbes take their vitamins because of how beneficial it is to the functioning of the immune system within the intestinal tract. And studies have found that grass-fed beef in particular contains beneficial amounts of omega-3 fatty acids, which are often lacking in the meat from conventional grain-fed cows.

SALMON 🄿 🄢 One of the most talked about power foods, salmon is rich in key health players omega-3 fatty acids and vitamin D, which can help normalize glucose levels via the gut. Salmon's other benefits include cardiovascular protection, improved mood and cognition, and joint health. Look for wild salmon from Alaska or Nova Scotia, or farm-raised salmon from countries such as Norway. To make an easy Wild Detox meal (or anytime meal, really), warm about a tablespoon of olive oil in a skillet over medium-high heat, season the fish lightly with a bit of salt, which naturally brings out the flavor in salmon, and then cook for 4 to 5 minutes on each side until the fish is cooked through and the flesh is flaky. Or, grill as you would chicken. (You'll also find a recipe for cooking salmon in parchment on page 166, which has the added bonus of leaving no pans to wash!)

SARDINES 🄿 🄢 are one of my top healthy protein choices. A serving of sardines provides more than 115 percent of the recommended daily intake of B_{12}, 70 percent of selenium, 43 percent of vitamin D, and, most notably, a hefty dose of omega-3s, which help protect the gut from intestinal inflammation. They are also economical and convenient to keep on hand or in your desk at the office because they are shelf-stable.

OTHER FISH AND SEAFOOD: COD, HALIBUT, SOLE, SCALLOPS, AND SHRIMP 🄿 🄢 All superior sources of protein, these fish are also rich in magnesium, which can improve mood and reduce anxiety thanks to the connection between our gut and our neurological system. They also contain omega-3 fatty acids; vitamins B_3, B_6, B_{12}; selenium; and phosphorus; and magnesium.

CHICKEN P L High in protein, chicken is extremely versatile and loaded with B vitamins, namely B3, which is like an energy source for your cells and plays a big role in your metabolic function, specifically the processing of fats and carbohydrates and even DNA synthesis.

Remember: Cooking any kind of meat at home is always a better option than buying it precooked. That roast chicken deli meat is convenient, but it's also likely loaded with nitrates and sodium; and whole roasted rotisserie chickens are typically full of sodium. There is really no reason to buy prepared chicken when it is so simple to cook it yourself: You can roast a whole chicken and use the meat for soups, stir-fries, salads, and sandwiches and make your own broth with the bones using the recipe on page 176. Alternatively you can cook a chicken breast by adding it to simmering water seasoned with fresh herbs and gently poaching over low heat, covered, for about 12 minutes. If you prefer the flavor of grilled chicken breasts, coat each side with olive oil and a pinch of salt, and then sear them in a grill pan over medium-high heat until cooked through, 4 to 6 minutes per side. Buying and cooking your own proteins also means you can be sure you are getting organic meat—and avoiding added hormones or antibiotics.

DRIED SEAWEED S A part of most seaside cultures' diets, seaweed contains prebiotic compounds, as well as a host of essential blood-building enzymes, vitamins, and minerals. A recent study has shown that eating sea vegetables—and the beneficial prebiotic fibers that come with them—is a boon for bacterial diversity in the gut. Plus, these vegetables taste like the ocean and make a delicious snack or addition to soups or salads. Dried seaweeds— including nori, hijiki, arame, and wakame—and can be found in most health food stores and in the Asian section of many markets. Be very careful when buying sea vegetables, though— source from a company that harvests from clean waters (or does third-party testing on the source waters) and regularly tests for heavy metals, herbicides, pesticides, and microbiological contaminants (see page 209).

MINERAL BROTHS P L S Both bone-based and vegetable-based broths are bursting with vitamins and minerals, and bone broths in particular are excellent guardians of gut health because their natural gelatin acts as a gut barrier protectant. This has been proven to be a useful attribute when it comes to healing gut health and reestablishing a healthy balance of flora.

I like to make my own from scratch and store the extras in the freezer. Store-bought broths are okay to use, but read the label for added sodium and preservatives. You'll find recipes for Mineral-Rich Bone Broth (page 176) and Roasted Vegetable Stock (page 174).

FERMENTED VEGETABLES P L S Fermented vegetables, such as cabbage, carrots, onions, and cucumbers, are one of the best ways to re-wild your gut. Most notably, they contain live cultures, such as lactobacillus, that help keep your gut populated with healthy flora. They also contain fiber and enzymes, which promote the growth of beneficial bacteria while also aiding digestion, as well as vitamin C. Note that fermented vegetables are not the same as pickles, which are preserved by means of an acidic solution without any fermentation. Try fermenting at home with this recipe.

CARROT AND CABBAGE KRAUT
Yield approximately 4 cups

I medium head cabbage, shredded

2 medium carrots, shredded

2 teaspoons fine Celtic sea salt

Spring water

In a medium bowl, combine the cabbage, carrots, and salt. Cover with a towel and leave to sit at room temperature for 30 minutes while the salt pulls juices out of the vegetables. Transfer to a wide-mouth quart jar or other fermenting container and cover the vegetables with spring water, leaving 1 inch of space at the top of the jar. Cover tightly with the lid or airlock. Leave at room temperature for 3 to 4 days and look for bubbles, which indicate the fermentation process has begun. In the first 24 hours, open the jar and press down firmly on the ingredients a few times to make sure they are fully submerged in the liquid. Taste the vegetables daily until they reach a consistency and flavor you like. At that point you should transfer your kraut to cold storage to slow the fermentation process. Fermentation is a continual process, so the flavor will change over time.

ALL VEGETABLES, ESPECIALLY DARK LEAFY GREENS P L S As much as I'd love to dedicate a paragraph to each and every vegetable under the sun, it would take up far too much space. Suffice it to say that these gems from the earth—when grown in healthy soil and without pesticides—are all fantastic for you. I'm particularly fond of leafy green vegetables, which protect the digestive and immune systems by strengthening the cells responsible for fighting infection and maintaining balance in the gut. A diet rich in cruciferous vegetables—kale, collard greens, broccoli, Brussels sprouts, cabbage—helps prevent cancer and other chronic diseases. Consider investing in a small electric steamer with a timer so you can toss vegetables in to cook while you prepare the rest of your meal. Otherwise, pour about 1 inch of water into a stainless steel vegetable steamer, add chopped vegetables, cover, and steam over medium heat until they're fork-tender, about 10 minutes.

SEA SALT **P** **L** **S** Unlike regular table salt, which is extracted from mines, heavily processed, and often treated with unnatural additives, a high-quality sea salt is unprocessed and loaded with minerals. (In my recipes I recommend Celtic Sea Salt brand, because the labeling of sea salt can be confusing.) At the start of your detox, I recommend dialing back your salt intake to allow your palate to readjust to the flavors of "real" foods, then gradually adding it back in to lightly season your food. You'll find that you don't need to rely on salt as much because plants and healthy animals pack so much flavor on their own, but when you do use it, use the good stuff.

WILD VINAIGRETTE **P** This is a Wild Detox essential because it offers great flavor that complements most plants while delivering beneficial fats. As I mentioned earlier, eating fats with plants helps the body assimilate the plants' nutrients so your body can more fully access all the good stuff they have to offer. Toss the vinaigrette (recipe on page 173) with lettuce and shredded veggies for a quick salad, drizzle it over roasted vegetables, or use it to marinate your meats or fish before cooking.

Honorable Mentions: Prebiotics

Eating probiotic-rich foods is important for keeping your gut wild, but they're more likely to flourish when you also ingest *prebiotic* fibers. As discussed earlier in the book, these foods are non-digestible carbohydrates, so they get safe passage through our GI tract and arrive intact to feed the beneficial critters in your gut. Get some of these prebiotic foods in each day:

ONIONS AND GARLIC 🅿 🇱 🆂 While you may not want to load up on either of these during a romantic date, adding them into your diet (especially raw) is well worth the halitosis. Onions and garlic are packed with inulin (the most common form of prebiotic), making them my top prebiotic pick.

Garlic in particular is a superstar. There are thousands of studies that demonstrate its antimicrobial, antiviral, and cancer-preventive benefits. My grandmother used to eat a few raw cloves a day (you read that right) and lived vibrantly until her late nineties. Garlic is one of the most powerful defenders against a weakened immune system and rampant viruses, which can result from dysbiosis and poor nutritional absorption.

ARTICHOKES 🅿 🇱 Artichokes contain fiber that has been directly linked to the growth of beneficial intestinal bacteria. While they are both different vegetables, the globe artichoke and Jerusalem artichoke (also known as sunchokes) are recognized as great sources of inulin, which can also increase your absorption rate for a variety of vitamins and minerals (especially calcium—your bones will thank you later).

DANDELION GREENS 🅿 🇱 These wild greens are a staple of the Greek diet. Some find them impossibly bitter to consume raw, but when you cook them down, the flavor mellows. That said, because cooking degrades some of the greens' nutrients, if you're feeling adventurous and want to rev up those "thin" microbes, aim for the stars and toss a raw handful into a salad. Plus, eating a bitter green raw means you can tell just how high its inflammation-busting polyphenol content is: The more bitter a green tastes, the more it's packing.

OATS 🅿 🇱 🆂 Oats are an ancient grain that can be traced back to the Fertile Crescent. In the digestive tract, fiber in oats ferments into short-chain fatty acids, which feed the intestinal microbes most responsible for keeping you lean. For an easy prebiotic burst, soak 1 cup rolled (not instant) oats overnight in coconut milk and you'll have a super-healthy breakfast waiting for you in the morning. Sprinkle with fresh berries and raw nuts, if you like.

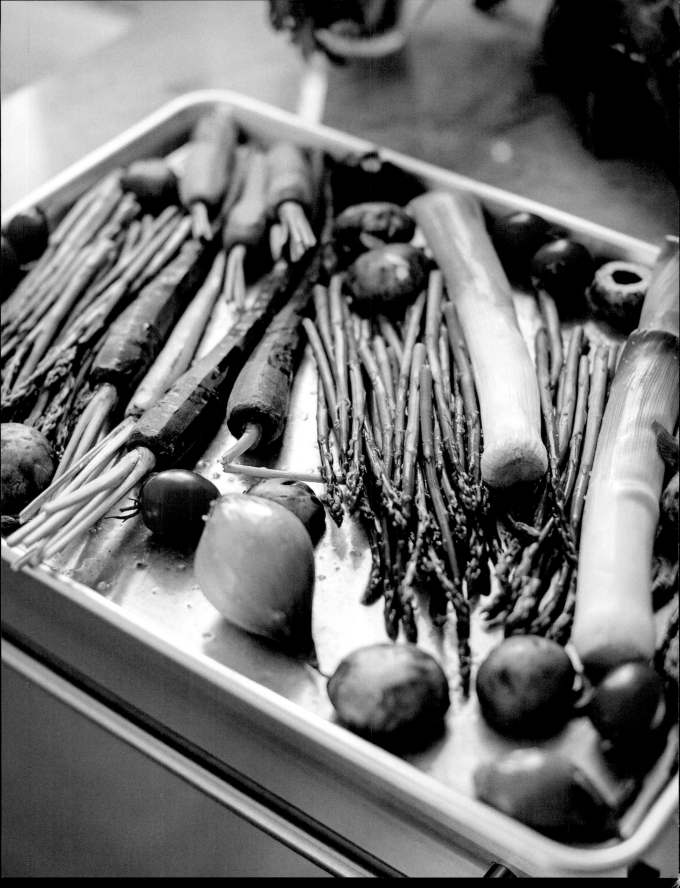

The Pre-tox

With your pantry fully loaded with the healthy, prebiotic, and nutrient-rich ingredients I've described, making Wild Pre-tox meals becomes a breeze. If you want to keep it super simple you don't even need to use a recipe, just combine two to four ingredients, being sure to include "one from the ground and one that makes a sound," otherwise, check out the recipes on pages 73 to 75. While these may not be chef-class meals that you would serve for a dinner party, you will find all of these easy combos tasty, satisfying, and most of all, effective. Some examples:

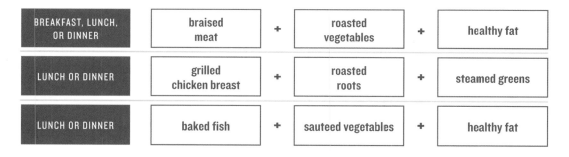

BREAKFAST, LUNCH, OR DINNER	braised meat	+	roasted vegetables	+	healthy fat
LUNCH OR DINNER	grilled chicken breast	+	roasted roots	+	steamed greens
LUNCH OR DINNER	baked fish	+	sauteed vegetables	+	healthy fat

Don't try to keep track of your calorie intake during the detox. Rather, I want you to focus on how to increase your daily intake of macronutrients, the major nutrients your body requires to perform basic functions. This way you'll be sure you're giving your body all the tools it needs to fuel, heal, and build.

• **HAVE UNLIMITED VEGETABLES.** Strive for at least 8 palm-size servings per day. Vegetables provide critical plant fiber, which ensures a healthy balance in your gut. By treating yourself to as many veggies as your heart—and belly—desire, you'll be getting plenty of nutrients while feeling fuller longer and boosting the gut microbes responsible for keeping you nice and lean. That said, you should pay close attention to your activity levels with regard to eating starchy carbohydrates like white potatoes, parsnips, plantains, green peas, and corn and avoid them on days when you have been sedentary. Don't forget to mix it up: roast diced butternut squash, mushrooms, and zucchini with some olive oil; or sauté green beans with garlic and sliced almonds. And aim to incorporate both raw and cooked veggies. Since you'll probably be eating more vegetables than you ever have—especially raw—they can, ahem, stop things up. Gently cooking or steaming vegetables helps your body break them down, access their nutrients, and keep things moving along smoothly in your digestive tract.

- **LET YOUR PALM GUIDE YOUR PROTEIN.** A simple way to determine a reasonable serving of protein is to use the size of your palm. (This is a good rule of thumb because our palms tend to be proportional to our overall frames, creating a customized yardstick for each individual.) Those who are moderately active can eat one palm-size serving of detox-approved protein. Double that if you are active, and triple if you're highly active. Generally speaking, moderately active means about 30 minutes of activity per day, whereas highly active means 90 minutes of activity or more.

- **PAIR PROTEIN AND VEGETABLES.** Anytime you eat protein, combine it with at least three servings of vegetables to help with digestion and to fortify the gut with beneficial plant fiber–producing bacteria. It also helps balance blood sugar, which is why—as you'll see in the sample detox on page 65—I recommend having protein and veggies any time of day. A serving of veggies is essentially the amount that could fit in your cupped palm. Bump it up to at least six servings if you are moderately active, and up to eight servings if you're very active. Again, as noted above, there really is no limit on the amount of healthful vegetables you eat, so if you are hungry, go for it!

- **CHOOSE YOUR FATS.** Wild-approved fats are a little trickier than the rest of the food strategy. Uncooked extra-virgin olive oil is always acceptable if you keep it to approximately 1 tablespoon per meal for moderate activity, 2 for active, and somewhere in between 2 or 3 for very active. You can also substitute other beneficial fats, such as grass-fed butter (like widely available brand Kerrygold) or coconut oil.

PRE-TOX AT A GLANCE

Here's what a day on the 3-day pre-tox might might look like:

UPON RISING

☐ Glucose Test

☐ 25 ounces of water

☐ Adaptogens (see page 46)

☐ Bee Pollen / Royal Jelly

☐ Whole Food Multivitamin

LIQUIDS ONLY UNTIL FIRST MEAL

☐ Yerba Mate (unsmoked)
OR
Peppermint and Chamomile Tea
(page 73)
OR
Organic coffee diluted with warm water

FIRST MEAL

☐ Dill Baked Salmon (page 75) with sweet
potato and ghee or butter

LUNCH

☐ Greek-Style Lemon Chicken (page 75)
with steamed vegetables and salad with
Wild Vinaigrette (page 173)

DINNER

☐ Rustic Vegetable Soup (page 75) OR
Stuffed Sweet Potato (page 74) with
Steamed Vegetables (page 74) and Wild
Vinaigrette (page 173)

I HOUR BEFORE BEDTIME

☐ ½ cup raw oats presoaked in ½ cup water
for 15 minutes

☐ Prebiotic supplement

☐ 8 ounces of water

Preparing to Land-Tox or Sea-Tox

With the three-day pre-tox behind you, it's time to move onto the next phase of the Wild Detox, the land-tox or sea-tox. Foodwise, this part of the program is very similar to the pre-tox in that you're aiming to eat lots of veggies plus lean proteins. The main difference is that I've added intermittent fasting (meaning you abstain from consuming *anything* except detox-approved beverages such as water and tea) from about 7 p.m. until 11 a.m. or noon the following day (roughly seventeen hours). Intermittent fasting helps balance your microbiome by essentially starving the bad bacteria in your gut, and can improve insulin sensitivity, stem cell and organ function, and resistance to stress. And by boosting gut health, fasting also helps enhance the immune system, and subsequently might help the microbiome prevent cancers from forming.

Because this is such a significant part of the program, I don't insist that you be as rigid about the proportions of nutrients you eat or how much water you drink as you were during the pre-tox. If you're feeling ravenous after your fast, go ahead and have more protein or healthy fats. If you're not strict about observing a 3:1 ratio of veggies to protein, I'm not going to report you to the detox police. The only thing I do ask is that you pay close attention to the detox-specific foods that you eat and supplements you take. This is because the particular foods I'm recommending for each program are crucial for helping you get "back to the wild," based on which of your body's systems are in the most need.

To determine which detox is best for you, take the quiz on page 67. Again, don't worry if it's not entirely clear which suits you best—your body will reap enormous benefits from going through either process. I've found, though, that most people tend to fall squarely into one category or the other. Once you know which detox you'll be following, refer to the detox-friendly foods on page 54 and note the ones specified for your program. Then all you have left to do is read up on the supplements I'm recommending (page 68) and look forward to how great you're going to feel.

QUIZ: SHOULD I LAND-TOX OR SEA-TOX?

Review both columns and put a check next to all the symptoms that apply to you. Whichever column has the most checks indicates which program you should follow.

LAND-TOX

- ☐ Feeling that bowels do not empty completely
- ☐ Hard, dry, or small stool
- ☐ Coated tongue or fuzzy debris on tongue
- ☐ Pass large amount of foul-smelling gas
- ☐ Burping
- ☐ Heartburn
- ☐ Irritable if meals are missed
- ☐ Cannot fall asleep
- ☐ Perspire easily
- ☐ Under high amounts of stress
- ☐ Insomnia
- ☐ Night sweats
- ☐ Fatigue after meals
- ☐ Must have sweets after meals
- ☐ Gain weight easily
- ☐ Overweight and/or puffy
- ☐ Acne

SEA-TOX

- ☐ Difficult, infrequent bowel movements
- ☐ Crave sweets during the day
- ☐ Depend on coffee to get you started
- ☐ Get lightheaded if meals are missed
- ☐ Eating relieves fatigue
- ☐ Poor memory, forgetful
- ☐ Blurred vision
- ☐ Roughage and fiber cause constipation
- ☐ Frequent urination
- ☐ Increased thirst and appetite
- ☐ Difficulty losing weight
- ☐ Tired, sluggish
- ☐ Feel cold: hands, feet, all over
- ☐ Require excessive amounts of sleep to function properly
- ☐ Increase in weight gain even with a low-calorie diet
- ☐ Depression, lack of motivation
- ☐ Morning headaches that wear off as the day progresses
- ☐ Dryness of skin and/or scalp
- ☐ Crave salt
- ☐ Weak nails

Your Land-Tox/Sea-Tox Supplements

Add these to your regimen along with those you took during your three-day pre-tox:

For the Sea-Tox

- **SEAWEED**: As discussed on page 58, sea vegetables are one of my secret weapons for getting people *really* healthy because they're loaded with benefits that heal the entire body. Seaweed is naturally antifungal, which helps protect the microbiome from overgrowth of damaging pathogens, particularly yeast. It's antibiotic, anti-inflammatory, and antioxidant, with studies suggesting it may inhibit tumor growth. And as an added bonus, it acts like a prebiotic, which in turn helps maintain balance in the gut and quiet an over-reactive immune system. I buy mine from Maine Coast Sea Vegetables (www.seaveg.com).

- **FISH OIL**: This magical supplement has been proven to help with weight loss, improve fertility, increase your energy, and give your skin a healthy glow. This is mainly because fish oil is one of nature's richest sources of omega-3 fatty acids. The sea-tox program will have you loading up on foods rich in omega-3s, but because fish oil has numerous benefits, I like making certain that you're getting every last bit that your body can use. I use either Carlson or Green Pasture brands.

  + If you experience "fish burps" when taking a fish oil supplement, try a smaller dose.

For the Land-Tox

- **MCT OIL**: MCTs—or medium-chain triglycerides—are actually a form of saturated fat. But before you dismiss them as a recipe for poor heart health, know that saturated fatty acids (think coconuts!) have a number of health benefits, including improved cognitive function, reduced body fat, and a more efficient immune system. If you cut healthy fats out of your diet in favor of carbohydrates, you will rob your body of one of the most crucial macro-nutrients you can get, and it's one that's missing from a lot of standard Western diets. The land-tox will help reintroduce healthy, unprocessed fats into your diet, but a supplement also will go a long way toward rebuilding your stores. I like Nature's Way Liquid Coconut Oil (www.naturesway.com) and Now Foods MCT Oil (www.nowfoods.com).

Here's a sample of what a day on your detox will look like, whether you are on a land-tox or sea-tox. Follow this template, mixing up the vegetables and proteins for three full days.

Land-Tox

☐ Intermittent fasting from 7 p.m. until 11 a.m. or noon, which can include drinking fast-friendly beverages: either yerba maté (unsmoked) or organic coffee mixed with hot water and 1 teaspoon coconut oil or butter

LUNCH (or whichever is your first meal after the fast)

☐ Supplements (one dose of each, per manufacturer's instructions)

☐ Land-tox–approved protein plus steamed or raw vegetables with Wild Vinaigrette (page 173)

DINNER

☐ Detox soup; the options include recipes for Italian-Style Turkey 'n' Onion Soup (page 74) and Rustic Vegetable Soup (page 75)

☐ Protein plus steamed vegetables with Wild Vinaigrette (page 173)

BEDTIME

☐ Mineral spray

☐ Prebiotic fiber supplement

☐ ½ cup raw rolled oats soaked in an equal amount of water for 5 minutes

Sea-Tox

☐ Intermittent fasting from 7 p.m. until 11 a.m. or noon, which can include drinking fast-friendly beverages: either yerba maté (unsmoked) or organic coffee mixed with hot water and 1 teaspoon coconut oil or butter

LUNCH (or whichever is your first meal after the fast)

☐ Supplements (one dose of each, per manufacturer's instructions)

☐ Miso soup or broth with seaweed plus Fresh Salad (page 73) with Wild Vinaigrette (page 173) OR Baked fish such as Fish Baked in Parchment (page 166) with dried nori and brown rice

DINNER

☐ Miso soup or broth

☐ Steamed fish and vegetables with nori sprinkles

BEDTIME

☐ Mineral spray

☐ Prebiotic fiber supplement

☐ ½ cup raw rolled oats soaked in an equal amount of water for 5 minutes

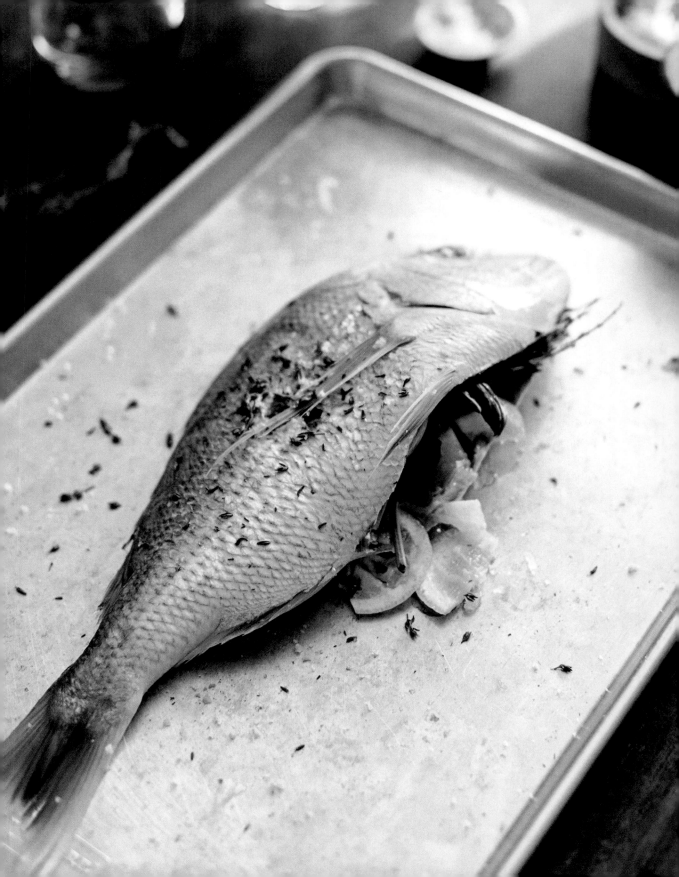

Detox Recipes

On pages 73 to 75, you'll find a few recipes that are representative of the type of food pairings I've found to be effective for facilitating a pre-tox or a land-tox/sea-tox. You can draw from this section when creating meal plans for your pre-tox plan (page 65) or your land-tox/sea-tox (page 69), or to create simple whole-food meals following the meal-planning guidelines on page 63. In most cases I recommend boiling and steaming over roasting because these cooking methods help thin out the cell walls of the vegetables and begin to metabolize the starch content, which enhances the bioavailability of their nutrients and makes them easier to digest.

Make a big batch of some (or all!) of these before beginning your detox, so you always have something delicious, healthy, and satisfying on hand.

TIPS FOR A SUCCESSFUL DETOX

- Keep fluids like water or peppermint tea with you at all times. Drinking water helps keep the body hydrated, which is particularly helpful when you're eating such a large amount of gut-scrubbing plant fibers. I think of drinking water as taking another supplement because of its health-boosting abilities. Including the specific amounts I recommend drinking throughout the day (upon rising, I hour before bed), aim for 3 liters of filtered water or spring water from a responsible source (I like Acqua Panna). The moment you feel a headache or lethargy—drink fluids.

- Feel free to snack: Any of the foods I recommend during the detox can be eaten in smaller quantities between meals. Aim for about one-fourth to one-fifth of what you'd eat for a full meal.

- Preparation is key: If you're not planning and preparing, you won't be able to fully commit. Take the time to clean out your kitchen and stock your fridge and pantry with everything you need. As you adjust to a new regimen you don't want to spend a lot of time figuring out what you're going to eat and where to get it. Many of my clients find they're most successful when they make a big batch of detox-approved meals on the Sunday before they begin and eat those prepared foods throughout the week.

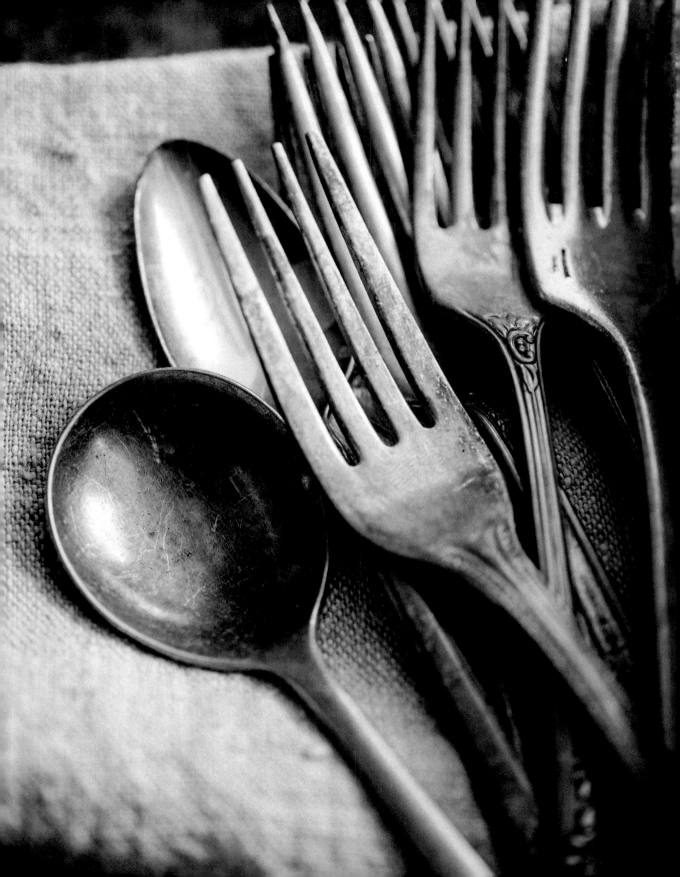

LAVENDER LEMONADE TONIC

Serves 2 to 4

l cup spring water

l tablespoon dried organic lavender or ¼ cup
fresh lavender blossoms, crushed

l bottle (750 ml) sparkling mineral water (such
as Gerolsteiner)

Juice of l medium organic lemon

l teaspoon maple syrup (optional)

Ice cubes, for serving

In a medium pot, bring the spring water to
a boil. Add the lavender and boil gently for
2 to 3 minutes. Strain into a bowl and set
aside to cool.

Transfer the lavender water to a large
pitcher. Add the mineral water, lemon
juice, and maple syrup (if using), mix well,
and refrigerate. Serve over ice.

PEPPERMINT AND CHAMOMILE TEA

Serves 2 to 4

8 cups spring water

5 peppermint tea bags

5 chamomile tea bags

Bring the water to a boil and pour into a
large heatproof bowl. Add the tea bags and
steep for 10 minutes. Discard the tea bags.
Store the tea in the refrigerator and either
drink cold or reheat.

FRESH SALAD

Serves 2 to 4

6 cups shredded greens

2 tablespoons extra-virgin olive oil

Juice of l lemon

2 tablespoons raw pumpkin seeds

Celtic sea salt, to taste

Toss everything together in a bowl and
refrigerate.

BERRY AND CHICKEN SALAD

Serves 2 to 4

3 cups shredded cabbage

2 cups chopped romaine lettuce

½ cup thinly sliced red onion

2 handfuls fresh berries

8 ounces cooked chicken breast, cubed

2 tablespoons extra-virgin olive oil

Pinch of Celtic sea salt

Combine all the ingredients in a large bowl
and toss together. Cover and store in the
fridge for up to 3 days.

STEAMED VEGETABLES

Broccoli, carrots, Swiss chard, or any vegetable you prefer (though starchier vegetables like potatoes, turnips, parsnips, etc., should be eaten in moderation), coarsely chopped

Fresh lemon juice

Celtic sea salt

In a steamer, steam the vegetables over boiling water until tender, about 8 minutes for most dense vegetables, 3 to 4 minutes for more delicate vegetables and greens.

Season with lemon juice, olive oil, and sea salt to taste. Store in the refrigerator for up to 4 days.

STUFFED SWEET POTATO

Serves 2

2 sweet potatoes, halved lengthwise

2 tablespoons extra-virgin olive oil

1 cup shredded cabbage

8 ounces cooked turkey or Greek-Style Lemon Chicken (page 75), shredded

Pinch of Celtic sea salt

Preheat the oven to 350°F.

Lay the sweet potato halves cut-side up on a baking sheet, brush lightly with olive oil. Bake until fork-tender, about 25 minutes.

Stack the cabbage and turkey on top. Season with olive oil and sea salt.

ITALIAN-STYLE TURKEY 'N' ONION SOUP

Serves 2 to 4

1 tablespoon extra-virgin olive oil

1 medium onion, chopped

3 garlic cloves, minced

5 cups Mineral-Rich Bone Broth (page 176) or store-bought bone broth or low-sodium chicken stock

2 cups water

½ cup chopped fresh flat-leaf parsley

2 cups shredded baked turkey or chicken (see Braised Turkey Breast recipe on page 154)

In a large saucepan, heat the olive oil over medium heat. Add the onion and garlic and sauté until softened, 5 to 7 minutes.

Add the broth and water and bring to a boil. Reduce to a simmer, add the parsley and shredded turkey, cover, and cook for 20 minutes.

Cool to room temperature and store in the fridge for up to 1 week.

RUSTIC VEGETABLE SOUP

Serves 2 to 4

I tablespoon extra-virgin olive oil
I medium yellow onion, diced
2 garlic cloves, minced
2 medium zucchini, diced
I cup shredded kale leaves or
   any other greens you prefer
10 mushrooms, chopped
I teaspoon dried rosemary
I teaspoon dried thyme
I teaspoon ground cinnamon
4 cups low-sodium chicken broth
Celtic sea salt and freshly ground black pepper

In a large soup pot, heat the oil over medium-high heat. Add the onion and sauté until translucent for 2 to 3 minutes. Add the garlic and sauté until golden brown, about 1 minute.

Stir in the zucchini, kale, mushrooms, rosemary, thyme, cinnamon, and broth. Bring to a simmer and cook until the vegetables are soft and cooked through, about 20 minutes. Season with salt and pepper to taste.

GREEK-STYLE LEMON CHICKEN

Serves 2 to 4

4 boneless chicken breasts
   (skinless if not organic)
Pinch of Celtic sea salt
I tablespoon dried oregano
I lemon, thinly sliced
2 tablespoons extra-virgin olive oil

Preheat the oven to 350°F.

Lay the breasts in a single layer in a baking dish and season with the salt and oregano. Top with the lemon slices and drizzle with the oil. Bake until cooked through, about 25 minutes.

Cover and store in the refrigerator for up to 1 week.

DILL BAKED SALMON

Serves 1

I (4- to 6-ounce) skinless salmon fillet
I tablespoon dried dill
Celtic sea salt
Extra-virgin olive oil

Preheat the oven to 350°F.

Lay the salmon in a baking dish. Season with the dill and sea salt to taste. Drizzle with olive oil and bake until cooked through, about 15 minutes. Serve warm, chilled, or at room temperature.

Coming Out of a Detox

Once you've completed whichever of the two Wild Detoxes you've chosen, you can begin to reintroduce foods into your diet, namely the Finicky Five: eggs, dairy, gluten, unprocessed soy, and corn. But don't just revert to your former diet! As you'll see in the next chapter, I recommend specific versions of these foods found in the Mediterranean diet. I also recommend that you add one new food every other day and then pay attention to how you feel after eating it. For example, if you notice bloating, remove the food from your diet immediately. If you're without any symptoms, you can continue to eat that food. Add the following foods in this sequence:

Days 1–2: Eggs

Days 3–4: Dairy

Days 5–6: Gluten (from whole-grain sources only)

Days 7–8: Corn

Days 9–10: Unprocessed Soy

After this, every three days you can reintroduce another of the foods you typically ate, one at a time, noting any symptoms that occur. If you feel that any of the foods reintroduced are causing your digestive system any trouble, go back to the Wild Detox meal plan.

The surest way to preserve the renewed, reinvigorated feeling you'll have after detoxing is to continue to make Wild Mediterranean foods the foundation of your diet. Instead of fixating on the foods that you might be eliminating, think instead about all the incredible flavors you'll be adding *in*. This way of eating is rich, flavorful, and satisfying—and takes little effort to source and to prepare. In the next chapter I'll explain how to "wild" your kitchen, including a full rundown of my favorite ingredients. And in Chapter 4, I've given you some of my favorite recipes from Mediterranean destinations that are known for their delicious and healthful fare—Greece, Italy, Spain, and France. These dishes will hopefully give you the inspiration you need to transform these foods from a *diet* into a *lifestyle*, while revitalizing the wild landscape of your digestive system.

Q. Will I experience any kind of symptoms during my detox?

A. It's very likely that you will experience mild discomfort at the beginning of your detox, especially on day two as your body begins to let go of the toxins it's been storing. You may feel fatigued, irritable, or foggy. Know that this will subside in about three days, at which point most of my clients report feeling measurably less bloated (including in places they didn't even know they had bloating, like their feet and hands), they'll urinate more owing to less water retention, their bowel movements become more productive, and they'll sleep better. So unless your discomfort becomes a true medical issue, my advice is to push through any symptoms and allow your body to heal.

Q. Should I exercise during the detox?

A. *Movement* during your detox is key. I don't mean setting aside 30 minutes to get your heart rate up to 160 beats a minute, I mean getting in gentle movement throughout the entire day—especially if you sit at a desk. Aim for at least 10,000 steps a day. We'll look more at the benefits of exercise in the next chapter, but basically, the gut requires circulation, just like the blood. So to really detox effectively, getting in regular movement is essential. And if you can also throw in some yoga or another fitness activity, go for it!

Q. I don't like some of the ingredients on the list, can I substitute with other foods?

A. No. That said, you don't have to consume an ingredient if it's not your favorite food item; you can omit and double up on another ingredient you prefer. Just don't add ingredients to the list.

Q. I don't have a refrigerator at work. How do I travel with the foods I've made?

A. No problem! An insulated lunch bag and a reusable ice pack should do the trick.

Q. What happens if I get super hungry?

A. This is probably the most common question I'm asked. It's simple: Consume more food from the approved ingredient list. Remember, there is no calorie count associated with the Wild Detox. What you'll most likely experience is your mind telling you you're hungry because it misses the foods you used to give your body—especially processed sugars and greasy, fatty foods. The brain is wired to want those things. But by giving yourself license to eat as much of the wild foods as you want, there's no way you'll be hungry.

Q. I have a social engagement that will require eating at a dinner with foods not on the plan. Will this impact all my efforts?

A. I ask that you schedule the cleanse during a time that you can commit 100 percent. So no foods that aren't on the list for those six days of pre-tox and detox.

Q. How are you feeling?

A. If you're not sure, revisit the quiz on page 41. If you score 3 or higher, you should consider a detox regimen every other month. If you feel your body needs another boost, consider a land- or sea-tox.

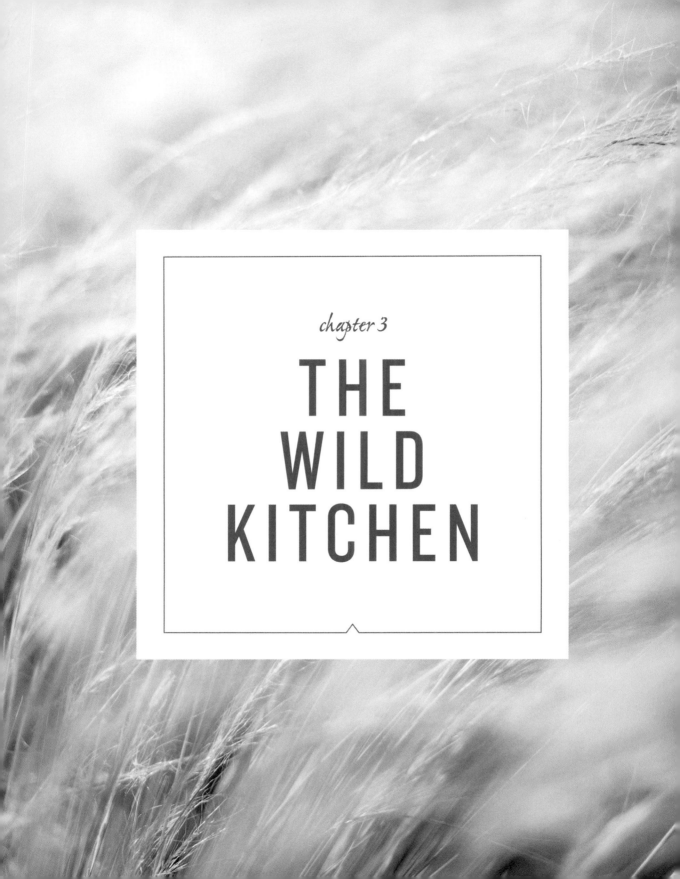

chapter 3

THE WILD KITCHEN

"Cooking and shopping for food brings rhythm and meaning to our lives."

Alice Waters

NOW THAT YOU'RE PREPARING TO TRANSITION FROM YOUR DETOX INTO "EVERYDAY LIFE," I WANT to introduce you to all the foods that make up the Wild Mediterranean diet—a diverse, delicious array of satisfying, nourishing foods for what I like to call eating "village-to-table." As is the case with the Wild Mediterranean lifestyle in general, eating wild isn't just about *what* to eat but also about *how* to eat it. That's because while from-the-earth, nourishing foods are absolutely the foundation for better health, so is finding joy and community. And there's no better way to do that than to do it with food—something Mediterranean villagers know a thing or two about. That's why after I'm done walking you through all the delicious new foods that will become the foundation of your new lifestyle, I'll introduce you to a concept that makes this new way of living so much more than a diet. It's called "finding your food tribe," and it's what makes the difference between trudging through a high-concept, fad program (I'm looking at you, Paleo!) and creating long-lasting change that's rooted in the kind of life you truly want to be living. So with that, on to the food!

The Wild Mediterranean kitchen has four basic components: fruits, vegetables, lean proteins, and unprocessed dairy (as well as some grains, on occasion). To help you find as much variety within these categories, I've added a go-to list of pantry and freezer essentials, which also includes a sampling of healthy fats, condiments, seasonings, and herbs. So get to the grocery store or farmers' market and go wild! And if you're in need of some inspiration for how to use these gut-curing staples, I've provided more than fifty recipes showcasing the many wonders of Wild Mediterranean foods, including their incredible power to diversify your gut with health-promoting bacteria and keep it balanced for the long haul.

Buying Wild

Plants

There's no better friend to your body than plant foods—particularly fruits and vegetables. They're packed with vitamins and minerals, aid digestion, boost the immune system, strengthen the nervous system, fortify the blood, and even prevent cancer. There's also no better friend to your gut than fiber, and these guys are packed with the stuff. Fiber nourishes our cells and reduces inflammation; and healthy microbes *love* getting their fill of it. Want to show your gut some TLC? Eat some plants! Making a habit of consuming a spectrum of fruits and vegetables, from apples to zucchini, diversifies the good bacteria in your gut, keeps you lean, and most important, keeps you satisfied. There's nothing more filling than a heaping bowl full of plant fiber. Nuts, seeds, and grains are also examples of super-powered plants, and we'll talk more about them later in this chapter.

When buying fruits and vegetables, I strongly recommend buying organic produce when you can find and afford it. The pesticides used to grow conventional produce can wreak havoc on your gut health by decimating the beneficial bacteria that live there, causing body-wide inflammation. Buying seasonally can help reduce the cost of organic produce as it's not being shipped from another continent. Eating food as it's coming up from the ground means you're reaping the most health benefits, plus there's no contest when it comes to taste. Exhibit A: Compare a perfumed, juicy, sun-ripened tomato from your garden or the farmers' market in August to a pale, mealy one from the store in December. And if your fruits and veggies taste better, I guarantee you'll eat more of them! Frozen organic fruits and vegetables offer another great option, as these foods are flash-frozen right after harvest. Often the frozen option is fresher than any nonlocal variety in the produce section that may have spent days if not weeks in a truck, or was picked too early so that it ripens on its journey.

If buying organic is absolutely not an option for you, consider limiting your purchases to foods not found on the Dirty Dozen; list compiled by the Environmental Working Group (www.ewg.org). These foods are the most heavily sprayed with pesticides and have thin skins that absorb said chemicals, and include strawberries, apples, nectarines, peaches, celery, grapes, cherries, spinach, tomatoes, sweet bell peppers (all colors), cherry tomatoes, and cucumber.

Vegetables

While I wouldn't single out any vegetable as being *un*healthy, I will advise you to be mindful of how much you eat of certain starchier vegetables, especially if you aren't active. These include corn, white potatoes, beans, peas, plantains, yucca, and taro. Here's a list of your *best* choices to give you some plant-spiration:

- ☐ Artichokes
- ☐ Avocados
- ☐ Broccoli
- ☐ Brussels sprouts
- ☐ Carrots
- ☐ Cauliflower
- ☐ Eggplant
- ☐ Fennel
- ☐ Garlic
- ☐ Leafy greens, such as kale, spinach, Swiss chard, and all lettuces
- ☐ Leeks
- ☐ Mushrooms
- ☐ Onions
- ☐ Radishes
- ☐ Scallions

Fruit

Fruit—especially citrus—is a key element in Mediterranean cuisine. Daily intake of some fruits, such as apples or pears or grapefruit—all rich in polyphenols—can significantly reduce body weight in obese people, and—you guessed it—help keep healthy bacteria in the gut flourishing. That said, I do recommend that you initially go easy on fruit as you transition to the Wild Mediterranean lifestyle. As healthy as fruit can be, it's still technically a "sugar," which can trigger you to want other unhealthy, sugary foods. If you're moderately active, stick to two servings a day. And of course, as is the case for all plant foods, be sure to choose fruit that is in season for optimal nutrition and flavor.

For citrus at its best, store it at room temperature. Great fruit options include:

- ☐ Apples
- ☐ Berries
- ☐ Figs
- ☐ Grapefruit
- ☐ Lemons
- ☐ Limes
- ☐ Oranges
- ☐ Peaches
- ☐ Pomegranates
- ☐ Watermelon

THE NITTY-GRITTY ON GRAINS

You'll notice that I don't include a lot of grains in the Wild Mediterranean diet, and it's for good reason. We've come a long way from the old-school food pyramid—the one whose base is loaded up with bread and pasta and rice and crackers—and the outdated recommendation that cereal is the cornerstone of a complete breakfast. Plus, processed foods—and refined grains like cereals, breads, and muffins are, indeed, processed foods—are no good for the gut. It's not that grains are necessarily bad, it's just that how we grow and manufacture goods made with them has changed for the worse.

We humans began harvesting grain about twelve thousand years ago, which ensured our ancestors a steady food supply. The good news was that our population exploded. The bad news was that this grain-focused diet caused the first widespread occurrences of food-related disease, because grains are proportionately lower in nutrients than food from animals or from most vegetables.

Another reason for the health downgrade among our forebears was that they had shifted away from wild ways of eating—the classic hunter-gatherer diet of bugs, seasonal vegetables, fruits, and nuts, supplemented by moderate amounts of meat and fish—and it happened in a short period of time. When they started farming grains, and had a regular and ready food supply, they ate fewer vegetables, and probably less meat, and that's where their nutritional troubles began.

In a way, we're in the same fix today. But our problem is in many ways worse because the grains we're eating—and the ultra-processed products derived from them—aren't grown using traditional methods. Rather, modern grain farming involves techniques such as dousing crops with pesticides and employing genetically modified (GM) seeds in order to increase crop yield and boost the bottom line for farmers and manufacturers.

It's no coincidence that the spike in gluten intolerance coincides with the increasing prevalence of such growing methods. Even for those who don't suffer from celiac disease, an autoimmune disorder, processed wheat can cause similar issues, including nausea, diarrhea, skin rashes, anemia, and even depression.

I always suspected there was something more to gluten intolerance than just the gluten, and I was right: Recent studies claim the use of glyphosate—one of the most widely used herbicides in the world—is the most important causal factor in the epidemic of celiac disease. What's particularly disturbing is that the majority of conventional wheat is grown from seeds that are genetically modified to withstand large amounts of glyphosate, allowing farmers to use even more of it on their crops. Farmers drench wheat crops with the herbicide in the field immediately prior to harvest because that actually kills the plant, which speeds the required drying time of the grain—a process known as "desiccation"—and offers a head start on killing off next year's weeds as a bonus. Researchers believe that, in some people, the glyphosate-treated wheat is what causes an imbalance in the small intestine, leading to the development of celiac disease. There's always a cost when you mess with Mother Nature. Maybe our microbiome is telling us something?

Whole grains traditionally include the three components of the grain: the bran (the fiber-rich outer layer), the germ (the nutrient-dense inner "nut" of the wheat), and the endosperm (the bulk of the kernel, containing a modest dose of vitamins and minerals). When all three parts are left intact, the wheat is referred to as "unrefined," and unrefined whole grains are considered a good source of fiber (although I believe plants are far superior in that regard). Refined or processed grains, on the other hand, are stripped of the bran and the germ, leaving only the endosperm. This provides a processed product with a smoother texture and longer shelf life. However, by removing those elements, much of the grain's nutritional value is lost. Food manufacturers will throw a bit of oat flour with inexpensive binders and fillers into a product so they can refer to it as "multi-grain," although there's really no additional health benefit—it just sounds good. You're still essentially taking in refined grains. Dr. David Ludwig—who has devoted his research to clearing up the carbohydrate confusion—warns that such a shift in our food supply will have detrimental effects for generations to come, citing that they're to blame for high levels of obesity in the very young and may eventually lead to the decrease in overall life expectancy.

While I'm certainly not anti-grain (I recommend having some rice and legumes on hand in the pantry, including wild rice—which is actually a grass!), I do recommend that you steer clear of their processed or nonorganic counterparts. You'll see in Chapter 5 that my flour-based recipes all call for *sprouted* wheat flour. This means the grains have been soaked in water until they begin to grow sprouts before milling, making it a living food. This process decreases the presence of enzyme inhibitors—a grain's natural defense mechanism that keeps it from being digested by hungry passerby in the wild—thereby making more of the grain's nutrients available and digestible to you. Also, don't fear farro or other "ancient" grains such as barley, emmer, and wheat berries, which, when sprouted, are very nutrient-dense and more readily digestible.

I have found over years of testing reactions to gluten-based foods with clients that about 80 percent of those with gluten problems can tolerate sprouted flours and grains without serious issues. This, of course, is after we remove all gluten from their diets with a pre-tox and detox. The rest remain quite sensitive and end up having to distance themselves from all wheat products.

Fresh Herbs

Herbs are card-carrying members of the plant family. Along with adding freshness when sprinkled over olive oil–drizzled vegetables and braised meats, herbs pack a number of health benefits, from the antimicrobial properties found in rosemary and oregano that can overpower drug-resistant pathogens to parsley's ability to cleanse toxins from the body and regulate blood pressure. No real Mediterranean meal is complete without these herbs—I especially couldn't imagine my life without oregano! To store fresh herbs, wrap them loosely in a dampened paper towel and place them inside a reusable plastic bag; they will stay fresh for up to a week. Or better yet, grow a few small pots of herbs on your kitchen windowsill or in your garden. Then harvest as needed and add them to anything and everything!

☐ Basil   ☐ Rosemary

☐ Dill   ☐ Sage

☐ Flat-leaf parsley   ☐ Thyme

☐ Mint   ☐ Bay leaves

☐ Oregano

Proteins

I believe most people do well on a protein-rich Mediterranean diet because we humans (as mammals) naturally produce hydrochloric acid, which is our secret weapon for breaking down proteins and reaping all their nutritional benefits. Animal proteins in particular—or those derived from fish and meat—can help beneficial bacteria flourish, normalize glucose levels, and perform not-so-small miracles such as improving mood and boosting cognitive function. Furthermore, the Wild Mediterranean diet, which tends to be heavier on fish than on red meat, accounts for lower rates of death from all coronary and cardiovascular causes. As I outlined in Chapter 2, I recommend combining protein food with plant fiber (ideally in a 3:1 plant-to-meat ratio) because the combination allows gut bacteria to break down and process all of these beneficial nutrients more fully, which means a gentler experience for the digestive and immune systems and more health benefits for you.

When it comes to buying meat and fish, it's extremely important to do so responsibly. As for meat and poultry, I again encourage you always to buy organic. Organic standards ensure that the animals have not been administered antibiotics or hormones, and that their feed has not been treated with pesticides or herbicides (and is not genetically modified). It also means that the animals are generally happier because they have access to fresh air, sunlight, and pasture. And happy animals = healthy animals. Note, though, that organic does not mean "grass-fed." In the case of beef in particular—where it has been shown that animals fed grass are far healthier than those fed corn because of corn's nasty effect on their own microbiomes—it's important to ask your butcher what type of diet that animal received. The only exception to buying organic is if you're purchasing meat or poultry directly from the farmer. Many small farmers can't afford an organic certification because it's expensive and involves jumping through a lot of regulatory hoops. Many of these farmers nonetheless offer a product far superior to what you can find in the store. So if you go to a farmers' market, just ask the farmer how their animals were raised!

There are a few considerations to keep in mind regarding seafood and shellfish as well. The first is the presence of mercury, which thanks to industrial processes, has seeped into our oceanic food supply. Mercury can bioaccumulate, meaning that any mercury in one fish is transferred to the next fish that eats it—and so on. Mercury is bad news because it's highly toxic, especially to the central nervous system. As a rule of thumb when choosing fish, the smaller the better. That's because larger fish typically have lived longer and are higher up on the food chain, which means they have had lots of time to gobble up smaller fish and are now the repository of all the heavy metals *they* had. On the other hand, little fish and mollusks—such as sardines and scallops—haven't had a chance to accumulate as much in their tissues. Other good options include salmon, mussels, rainbow trout, mahi mahi, halibut, shrimp, and Atlantic mackerel.

> Combining protein with plant fiber allows gut bacteria to break down and process all of these beneficial nutrients more fully, which means a gentler experience for the digestive and immune systems and more health benefits for you.

I once had a client whose standard lab reports and GI test made him look pretty darn healthy on paper, yet he complained of frequent loose stools. It wasn't until I ran a urinalysis specifically for heavy metal toxicities that we found his levels were way above what's considered normal—his weekly ritual of swordfish tacos had been loading up his system with mercury. I told him to switch to well-sourced mahi mahi, halibut, or shrimp, and after retesting a month later, his mercury levels had gone down considerably.

The other thing to keep in mind when buying fish and shellfish is how sustainably it's being caught or farmed. Ideally you'd aim for seafood that's been raised with consideration for the long-term vitality of the species and the health of the lakes, rivers, and oceans. It will mean fewer antibiotics and better-quality feed for the fish, and in exchange, more nutrition for you.

The Wild Pantry, Fridge, and Freezer

Take a moment to inventory your refrigerator, cupboards, and freezer. Having a well-stocked pantry is the first step toward cooking nutrient-rich food. Ditch or donate any highly processed stuff lurking in your kitchen; you won't be eating it anymore, and you need to make room for all the nutrient-dense, gut-revitalizing food that will now form the core of your diet.

Dairy

About 65 percent of Americans have some level of lactose intolerance. That's one of the reasons I advocate removing all dairy during the pre-tox, sea-tox, and land-tox, and then adding it back to your regular diet mindfully. That said, some dairy products can be a real boon to digestive health, particularly fermented products such as yogurt or kefir. Aged cheese, a microbiologist's dream cocktail of beneficial bacteria and fungi, is also a great addition to the rotation. All those colonies of living critters interacting with one another over time are not only what give cheeses their character—the blue veins of Roquefort, bubble-dotted Swiss, the powdery rind of Brie—but also the probiotic power that your digestive system needs to thrive. It, along with other fermented or live-culture foods, is a perfect example of how eating wild is so far superior to taking a probiotic supplement for re-seeding the gut. Ten thousand years ago our ancestors may not have known what revolutionary science they were on to when making the first cheeses, but it's an excellent illustration of how ancient wisdom has found its way into our modern health.

When adding dairy back into your diet, pay attention to your system, and even consider doing some pre- and post-prandial glucose testing (page 51) to determine if the sugar in dairy impacts your insulin reaction. If it does, give goat milk a try. Goat's milk may help cut inflammation in the gut, which in turn protects your mucus membranes and boosts overall immune function. Eggs are another potentially immunogenic food, so be mindful when reintroducing them into your daily meals as well. When buying dairy, my guideline is simple: Buy organic.

- ☐ Feta cheese
- ☐ Ghee
- ☐ Goat milk
- ☐ Kefir
- ☐ Low-fat milk
- ☐ Low-fat yogurt
- ☐ Hard aged cheese (ideally sheep or goat varieties, preferably raw), such as Parmigiano, pecorino, Manchego, Zamorano, or Comté, just to name a few
- ☐ Ricotta cheese
- ☐ Eggs

Pantry, Fridge, and Freezer Staples

With these items on hand, there's always something to eat.

- ☐ Olives of all varieties
- ☐ Capers
- ☐ Canned fish, including anchovies, tuna, sardines, and salmon packed in oil
- ☐ Dijon mustard
- ☐ Artichoke hearts in oil
- ☐ Canned beans: cannellini, kidney, chickpeas (look for organic and BPA-free)
- ☐ Extra-virgin olive oil
- ☐ Dried lentils
- ☐ Rices, including long-grain, Valencia-style short-grain, and wild rice
- ☐ Canned tomatoes and tomato paste, with no added sugars
- ☐ Infused oils, such as chili oil
- ☐ Worcestershire sauce
- ☐ Dried fruits such as figs, prunes, and cranberries
- ☐ Nuts and seeds, including almonds, cashews, coconuts, pine nuts, pistachios, walnuts, and pumpkin and sunflower seeds.

- [ ] Vinegars, including apple cider vinegar, white wine and red wine, balsamic (more expensive balsamics don't contain added sugars)
- [ ] Coconut sugar
- [ ] Honey
- [ ] Sun-dried tomatoes
- [ ] Dried mushrooms, such as shiitake, chanterelles, and porcini
- [ ] Bay leaves, dried thyme, oregano, rosemary, sage, mixed Italian herbs
- [ ] Cayenne, ground cinnamon, ginger, cumin, paprika
- [ ] Red pepper flakes
- [ ] Fennel seeds

OLIVE OIL: THE ANCIENT SUPERFOOD

Olive oil has been a known digestive tonic for millennia. The Greeks were most likely the first to discover its remarkable health benefits, from use as digestive aid to a beauty product. Now modern science has confirmed that they were right: Consuming extra-virgin olive oil in particular has a number of health benefits, including anti-inflammatory qualities, the stabilization of insulin and blood sugar levels, and lower cholesterol. Olive oil is easily digested and readily absorbed by the body, and positively impacts every part of your digestive system. It can reduce both the risk of acid reflux and the potential for gallstones (thanks to the help it gives to the liver and pancreas in their daily functions). It also has a mild laxative effect, which helps combat constipation. Since antiquity, people have known about the benefits of consuming olive oil, which were attributed to its high oleic acid content. However, it is now well established that these effects can also be due to its antioxidant, anti-inflammatory, and antimicrobial powers.

You can and should use olive oil in dozens of ways. A bit of high-quality extra-virgin olive oil (EVOO) and a splash of lemon can perk up simple steamed or sautéed food, while a slick of virgin olive oil (VOO) will add flavor and moisture to roasted fish and vegetables. I even use it as a beauty product.

When buying olive oil, keep in mind that extra-virgin is made by a process called "first cold-pressed." The word *first* refers to the olives that are pressed the first time around and "cold" means that olives are not incubated in temperatures higher than 81.9°F. This type of processing ensures that no heat or chemical additives were used to extract the oil, and that the olive oil retains its full nutritional value. Opt for extra virgin over "pure" olive oil, which can be chemically processed, and "light" olive oil, which is a mix of virgin and processed oil. These oils lack the health benefits of EVOO.

Salt and Pepper

If you've gone through the Wild Detox, you will likely find that your taste preferences have changed and you may need little or no salt to appreciate vibrantly fresh food. Toss your highly processed white salt and pick up natural fleur de sel or Celtic sea salt. It will cost a bit more, but the flavor boost will be worth it, and you'll find yourself using less. Plus, you'll be reaping the benefits of lots of natural minerals. Freshly ground pepper also makes a world of difference in terms of flavor and culinary punch.

Eating Wild Doesn't Mean Spending Wildly

I know what you're thinking: *How can I afford all these fresh, organic foods and fancy olive oils and salts? And how on earth am I supposed to find time to whip up all these fancy meals?* Well, you can stop worrying. I know firsthand that the Wild Mediterranean diet is not only less expensive than your current diet but also is more efficient (and effective). There's even a study that backs me up. The Miriam Hospital and the Rhode Island Community Food Bank asked food bank clients to cook Mediterranean-inspired recipes three times a week. Their finding? Buying ingredients for meals based on fruits, veggies, and healthy fats—with smaller portions of lean meats—actually cost *$750 less per person per year* than the USDA's cheapest healthy recommendations. Best of all, the participants reported that not only were their groceries cheaper but they also spent less time preparing meals than they had previously. Most important, they felt much better physically, too.

Drink for Your Gut

A major study in The Netherlands found that drinking tea, wine, and coffee had a positive impact on the diversity of the microbiome. A moderate intake of wine provides beneficial antioxidant properties, glucose-balancing, and expanded biodiversity thanks to its suspected role as a prebiotic, although overindulgence will have a negative effect. (See "Alcohol," page 198.)

Both black and green tea have been shown to increase activity in the microbiota, although green tea appears to be particularly beneficial. Both aid nutrient absorption in the small intestine. Drinking coffee and tea can help you feel more satiated, and also consume less food and avoid snacking. Drinking black tea has also been associated with a reduced risk of cardiovascular disease. Green tea, rich in polyphenols, may play a role in weight loss. I always recommend buying organic coffee, wine, and tea. And I also have to offer the caveat that since everyone's gut is different, your reaction to various beverages will vary. If you find yourself hungry, irritable, or you feel like your blood sugar has spiked and crashed, consider doing pre- and post-prandial glucose testing as outlined in Chapter 3 to see if any particular category of beverage has a negative impact on your own levels of blood sugar.

Find Your Food Tribe

Bringing a bit of Greece back to Los Angeles with them, my father and his friends from Athens regularly head out for dinners at local Greek restaurants. They share a meal, argue passionately about things like which region of Greece produced the best olive oil, and stop to admire beautiful women passing by. They sit—sometimes for hours—sharing stories, sharing jokes, sharing hardships. I used to love going with him to these dinners, remembering the same spirit among fellow villagers on my trips to Greece.

> Something really special happens when you surround yourself with people who share your values about what you're putting in your body. After all, this isn't a diet. This is a way of life.

Aside from eating nourishing, whole foods, a crucial element of the Mediterranean lifestyle is finding your "food tribe." It's connecting with like-minded people who share your views on, quite simply, how to live a good life. This, of course, has a lot to do with what we eat, but also extends to things like healthy work-life balance, the importance of community, and a general worldview that feels compatible with and supportive of yours. Is it possible to find this kind of kinship with people who aren't specifically following a Mediterranean diet? Of course! But something really special happens when you surround yourself with people who share your values about what you're putting in your body. After all—as we've talked about from page 1—this isn't a diet. This is a way of life.

If you lived in Greece, Spain, France, or Italy, you'd naturally be surrounded by people who ate and lived like you. Now it takes a little effort to carve out that community—but not without great payoff. Finding your food tribe means tapping into a support system, a social network, and—essentially—your village. Creating this sense of camaraderie can be a significant source of joy in your life—which is excellent for your health.

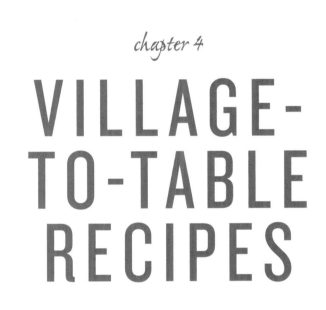

chapter 4

VILLAGE-TO-TABLE RECIPES

AS I'VE NOTED THROUGHOUT THIS BOOK, EATING "VILLAGE-TO-TABLE" IS THE KEY TO THE WILD Mediterranean lifestyle. It means calling upon the foods and cooking methods used for generations in countries like Greece, Spain, France, and Italy—and that have been the foundation for health in those communities. I'm focusing on these four countries here because the fundamental ingredients of those cuisines are not only healthful, they're also easy to find in most grocery stores. Many of the recipes in this book feature a "Four Countries, Four Ways" approach—one simple dish made in the styles of these four cooking traditions. You'll also see a number of recipes for familiar "comfort food" dishes—from French toast to risotto to meatballs—which I've made over to include more healthful, digestion-healing ingredients. These small tweaks aren't about feeling "guilt-free" or skimming on calories—in fact, I'm against any associations between guilt and food. The idea here is to create something really tasty that also supports happiness in the biome.

Ultimately, you'll start to recognize that cooking fresh, simple ingredients using basic methods is easy, delicious, and makes you feel great, too. That's because when you're eating across the food groups, you're doing a better job of nurturing your digestive system. The more diversity in your diet, the more diversity there will be in your gut. Instead of counting carbs or being a stickler about fat, focus on getting that ideal 3:1 vegetable-to-meat ratio, which these recipes support. So go ahead—eat your way to better health!

A NOTE ON INGREDIENTS

These recipes call for a few specific ingredients whose nutritional benefits I've outlined in Chapter 3. Please note that when possible all butter should be grass-fed (such as Kerrygold); oil should be high-quality (I've listed many of my favorites in the Resources section on page 209); salt should be unprocessed Celtic sea salt or fleur de sel; and eggs, proteins, and produce should be organic.

Unless specified otherwise, filtered water should be used for recipes that call for water.

BREAKFAST

—

One way to prepare the body and mind for the day is to start with a little creativity. In the village, meals are uncomplicated, most made from just a handful of ingredients, but I try to enliven things by combining ingredients in unexpected ways, like my Sprouted Cinnamon-Maple French Toast (page 99). For many of us, breakfast can be a rushed affair, hardly giving us a chance to appreciate what we're eating. Take the time to slow down and savor if you can, or just find a few minutes to sit and enjoy the morning sun with your tea. The ritual of enjoying the beginning of a new day is just as important as the meal itself.

DEEP-DISH FRITTATA

Butternut Squash · Mushroom · Scallion · Thyme

Serves 4

I small butternut squash (about I pound), peeled and cut into I½-inch cubes

I tablespoon extra-virgin olive oil, plus more for serving

Celtic sea salt and freshly ground black pepper

I tablespoon unsalted butter

I medium red onion, finely chopped

8 cremini mushrooms, trimmed and chopped

I teaspoon fresh thyme leaves

2 scallions, white and light green parts, diced, plus more for serving

6 eggs, lightly beaten

Shaved pecorino cheese, for serving

Mediterraneans keep their cooking low-fuss by using ingredients that are local and seasonal. This means they can reap the most flavor with little effort. This frittata is a perfect example of that: It's a simple technique that's also the ultimate canvas for showcasing fresh produce and herbs. You can always depend on this dish when you want to eat healthfully and quickly. Have a slice with a cold glass of white wine for a light summer supper.

wild bonus: Thyme contains antimicrobial properties that help protect the large intestine against not-so-friendly bacteria and pathogens.

Preheat the oven to 350°F. Lightly butter a 9-inch springform pan.

Place the butternut squash cubes on a baking sheet and lightly brush them with the olive oil. Bake until fork-tender and caramelized, about 25 minutes. Season the squash with salt and pepper to taste and set aside to cool. (Leave the oven on.)

Meanwhile, in a large skillet, heat the butter over medium-high heat. Add the onion and cook until softened, 5 to 7 minutes. Add the mushrooms and thyme and cook until the mushrooms are tender, another 1 to 2 minutes. Remove from the heat and allow the mixture to cool.

In a medium bowl, combine the scallions and eggs. Add the cooled squash and onion mixture and mix well.

Pour the contents of the bowl into the prepared springform pan. Bake the frittata until lightly browned on top, about 20 minutes. Top with pecorino, scallions, and olive oil to taste.

YIAYIA'S EGGS MATI

Oregano · Cracked Pepper

Serves 1 or 2

1 teaspoon unsalted
butter

2 eggs, preferably at
room temperature

1 tablespoon water

Pinch of Celtic sea salt

Dash of dried oregano

Drizzle of extra-virgin
olive oil

Pinch of coarse black
pepper (optional)

My grandmother always made sure we had our eggs sunny-side up, or *mati* (Greek for "eye"). Without knowing the science behind it, she always felt that the golden yolk contained a plethora of nutrients—especially B vitamins—that shouldn't be overcooked. As it turns out, she was right, so I recommend that you eat your eggs mostly *mati*. That said, fully cooked eggs are still loaded with nutritional benefits (tons of protein, healthy cholesterol, and choline, which is awesome for brain health).

This recipe involves two of my favorite egg secrets: Use a cast-iron pan, which not only distributes heat well but also infuses your food with trace (and healthy) amounts of iron, but also uses steam to cook eggs, so they turn out perfectly every time. Make sure your pan has a tight-fitting lid.

wild bonus: Egg yolks are a superior source of vitamin D, which helps keep the immune system in your microbiome functioning optimally.

In a small skillet, heat the butter over medium-high heat. Give the butter a swirl to assure that it coats the bottom of the pan well. Crack the eggs into the pan and add 1 tablespoon water. Cover with the lid, immediately reduce the heat to medium-low, and cook until the whites are set but the yolks remain runny, about 1 minute (or longer if you like a firmer egg). Use a spatula to transfer the eggs to a plate and season with the salt, oregano, olive oil, and pepper (if using).

SPROUTED "CREPES"

Ricotta · Berries · Maple

Serves 2

2 eggs

I teaspoon vanilla extract

2 sprouted-grain tortillas
(such as Food For
Life Ezekiel full-size
tortillas)

½ cup whole-milk ricotta
cheese

I tablespoon pure maple
syrup, plus more for
serving

I tablespoon unsalted
butter

Berries, for serving

You'll find a creperie on pretty much every commercial block in most southern Mediterranean countries. Crepes can be healthy—or totally decadent. This version is both! I wanted to make something easy and healthy at the same time that still scratches the itch for something indulgent and sweet.

Feel free to experiment with your own flavor combinations using this basic recipe.

wild bonus: Although it's still a "sugar," maple syrup contains something called phenolic compounds, which are believed to protect against cancer.

In a shallow bowl, beat together the eggs and vanilla with a whisk or fork. Soak the tortillas for 2 minutes in the egg mixture.

In a small bowl, whip together the ricotta cheese and maple syrup. Set aside.

In a large skillet, heat the butter over medium-high heat. Fry each egg-soaked tortilla until golden brown 1 to 2 minutes on each side.

Divide the ricotta filling between the "crepes." Fold the right and left sides of the crepe together, meeting at the middle and overlapping slightly. Now roll the bottom of the crepe up to the top. Finish with additional maple syrup if desired and fresh berries.

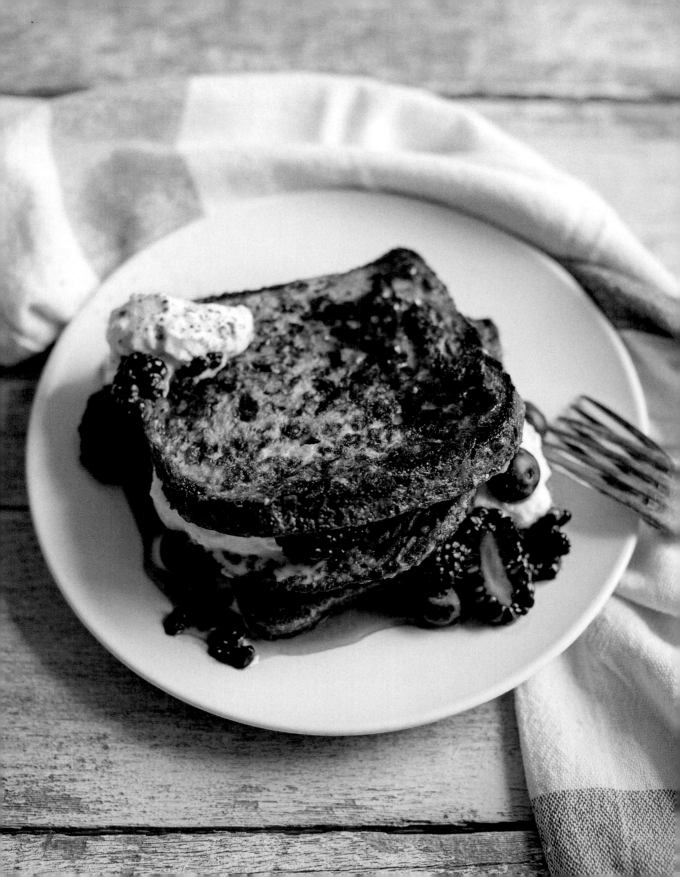

SPROUTED CINNAMON-MAPLE FRENCH TOAST

Cinnamon · Maple · Egg

Serves 2

2 eggs

½ cup unsweetened almond milk

I teaspoon ground cinnamon, plus more for sprinkling

I teaspoon vanilla extract

4 slices sprouted cinnamon raisin Ezekiel bread

I tablespoon unsalted butter

Maple syrup, for serving

Who doesn't love French toast? You'll particularly like this adaptation, which has the same classic flavors while getting in some fiber with the sprouted wheat and protein from the egg. This recipe is similar to the idea of the sprouted "crepe" (page 97)—taking a beloved comfort food and adding a gut-friendly twist.

wild bonus: You have a microbiome in your mouth—it's part of the digestive system, after all!—and studies have shown that cinnamon helps support it and prevent dental cavities.

In a shallow bowl, use a whisk or fork to whip together the eggs, almond milk, cinnamon, and vanilla. Soak the bread slices in the egg mixture for 2 minutes.

In a skillet, heat the butter over medium-high heat. Add the bread and cook until golden brown, 1 to 2 minutes on each side.

Serve the toast with maple syrup and a sprinkle of cinnamon.

SALADS & VEGETABLES

══

Wild Mediterranean is all about integrating the past with the present. So much of our food wisdom can be traced to earlier times, including the way we raise and consume vegetables. Eating locally grown vegetables in their natural seasons, patronizing farms and vendors known for the quality of their produce, and using just the right type of ingredient for what you're cooking: all of these things bring us closer to the rhythms that are instinctive to Mediterranean villages.

GRAPEFRUIT SALAD

Celery · Pistachio · Mint

Serves 4

3 Ruby Red grapefruits

I celery stalk, finely chopped

3 tablespoons pistachios, coarsely chopped

5 fresh mint leaves

Extra-virgin olive oil

Celtic sea salt

Citrus season in the US comes right in the nick of time during the cold, dreary months of winter and early spring when most people need to amp up their nutrient intake. I prefer Ruby Red grapefruit for this salad, and don't skimp on the olive oil—it's what really pulls the dish together.

wild bonus: Grapefruit contains an abundance or polyphenols, which help facilitate a beneficial balance of bacteria in the gut.

Peel and segment the grapefruits. Make sure all the pith is removed or it will taste bitter. Arrange the pieces neatly on a plate and sprinkle with the celery and pistachios. Tear the mint leaves and arrange them on top. Finish with a generous drizzle of olive oil and sea salt to taste.

ENDIVE SALAD FROM BEAUNE

Endive · Apple · Pear · Walnut Roquefort

Serves 2 as a main dish or 4 as a side

5 Belgian endive, cored, leaves separated

I handful baby greens

I apple, thinly sliced

I pear, thinly sliced

½ cup roughly chopped walnuts

4 tablespoons Wild Vinaigrette (page 173)

3 tablespoons crumbled Roquefort cheese

Celtic sea salt and freshly ground black pepper

In France, most of the salads you find in restaurants are ultra seasonal—they've really stayed true to the notion of eating with the seasons. This classic combination shows up on menus come fall. Endive is commonly used as a bitter green in Mediterranean cuisine, often balanced by something sweet, such as pear or apple. A crisp, tart apple works best here, such as a Honeycrisp or Granny Smith.

wild bonus: Fermented cheeses like Roquefort contain many different strains of probiotics, compared to the two or three strains found in most commercial "probiotic" yogurts.

In a large bowl, combine the endive leaves, baby greens, apple, pear, and walnuts. Drizzle on the dressing, add the Roquefort, and gently toss to coat. Season with salt and pepper to taste. Serve immediately.

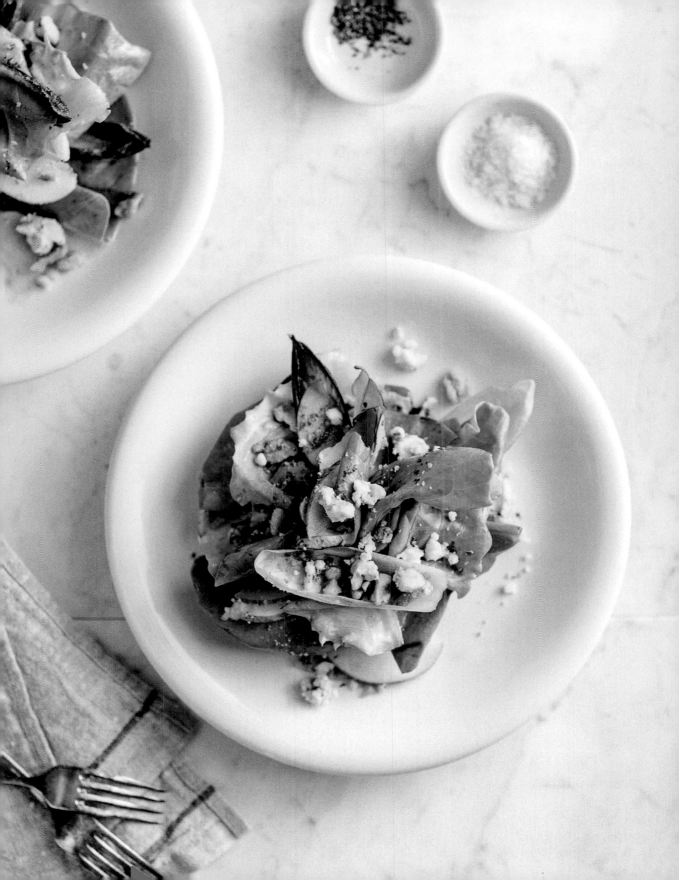

FRENCH-MEETS-GREEK SALAD

Carrots · Radicchio · Avocado · Feta

Serves 4

I head radicchio, cored and finely chopped

I fennel bulb, trimmed of stalks, cored, and finely chopped

I package (16 ounces) frozen heirloom Parisian carrots, thawed, or I pound organic carrots, sliced

I teaspoon unsalted butter

I teaspoon fresh thyme leaves or fresh basil, chopped

2 teaspoons Celtic sea salt

1½ teaspoons freshly ground black pepper

I can (15 ounces) chickpeas, drained and rinsed

5 tablespoons extra-virgin olive oil

2 tablespoons fresh lemon juice

I avocado, sliced

¼ cup crumbled feta cheese

This lovely layered salad makes use of Parisian heirloom carrots, more commonly referred to as Tonda di Parigi. That's right—carrots grown from heirloom seeds in France and Belgium with an Italian name. They're the size of a radish and, at first glance, look like tiny pumpkins. In addition to their unique look, they are also a particularly sweet carrot. You can usually find them in the frozen vegetable case at the grocery store. However, this dish is just as delicious with organic baby carrots, too.

wild bonus: An avocado a day keeps the doctor away. The monounsaturated fatty acids in avocados help boost beneficial flora in your gut, which ultimately leads to a stronger immune system.

Combine the radicchio and fennel in a large bowl. Set aside.

Leave the Parisian carrots whole, but if you're using a regular carrot, cut on an angle into ⅛-inch-thick slices.

In a large saucepan, heat the butter over medium heat. Add the carrots, thyme, 1 teaspoon of the salt, and pepper and gently sauté until the carrots have softened, about 3 minutes. Allow the carrots to cool before adding them to the salad bowl with the radicchio and fennel.

In a small bowl, combine the chickpeas, 3 tablespoons of the olive oil, the lemon juice, and the remaining salt and season with the pepper. Lightly mash the beans with a fork.

To serve, top the vegetable mixture with the chickpea mixture, avocado, and feta. Drizzle with the remaining 2 tablespoons olive oil and season with additional pepper if desired.

LUCCA-STYLE SALAD

Romaine · Carrot · Dill · Balsamic

Serves 2 as a main or 4 as a side salad

1 head romaine lettuce, finely shredded

6 medium carrots, finely shredded

3 tablespoons chopped fresh dill

1 tablespoon balsamic vinegar

3 tablespoons extra-virgin olive oil

Celtic sea salt and freshly ground black pepper

When you buy fresh foods at the peak of their seasonality, even the most basic ingredient can be deeply flavorful. This salad is the perfect representation of that.

wild bonus: Carrots contain properties that help increase the enzymes in saliva that aid in digestion.

In a medium serving bowl, combine the lettuce, carrots, and dill and mix well by hand. Top with the vinegar and olive oil, toss well, and season with salt and pepper to taste.

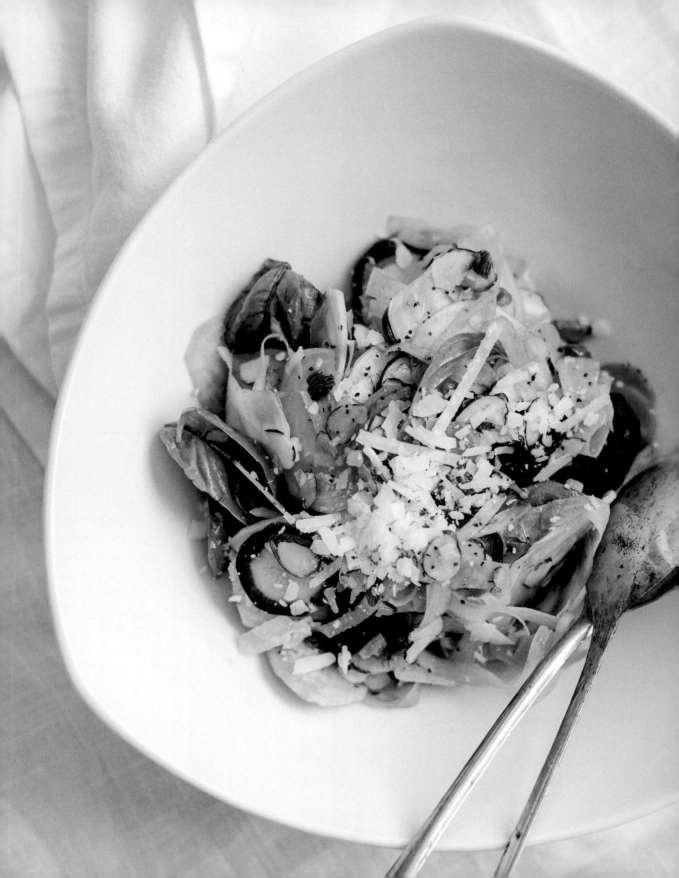

"ROOT-DOWN" SALAD

Beet · Sheep Cheese · Basil

Serves 4

For the Salad:

2 medium red beets, peeled

2 medium yellow beets, peeled

2 medium carrots, peeled

1 tablespoon extra-virgin olive oil

Pinch of Celtic sea salt

For the Nut Mixture:

3 tablespoons sliced almonds

Juice of 1 medium orange

1½ tablespoons extra-virgin olive oil

¼ cup grated hard sheep's cheese or crumbled soft goat cheese, such as chèvre

Remember the movie *Goodfellas,* where Paul Sorvino's character is slicing the garlic paper-thin? This raw root vegetable salad definitely benefits from the same treatment, which is why I recommend that you invest in a mandoline to make it. Slicing beets and carrots as thinly as possible gives them a sweeter, less "root-y" taste, which pairs perfectly with sheep's milk cheese and fresh basil.

This recipe is a fantastic opportunity to do what you want with a dish. If you like a bit more beet and less carrot, or want to add arugula, change up the cheese, or try walnuts or hazelnuts instead of almonds . . . that's the joy of cooking! You could even omit the dressing called for here and use Wild Vinaigrette (page 173) in its place.

wild bonus: Beets are loaded with fiber, which helps keep the mucous membranes in your gut healthy.

To make the salad: Using a mandoline or v-slicer, slice the beets and carrots paper-thin. Place the beets and carrots in a bowl and add the olive oil and salt. Toss and set aside.

To make the nut mixture: Place the almonds in a small bowl. Whisk in the orange juice and olive oil, mix well, and set aside.

To serve, arrange the beets and carrots in shallow dishes and top with the nut mixture. Add a sprinkle of your favorite sheep's milk cheese. Go cheese-heavy on this dish!

SUNCHOKE CHIPS

Serves 4 to 6

I pound small Jerusalem artichokes (sunchokes)

½ teaspoon Celtic sea salt

Grated zest of I unwaxed lemon

I tablespoon finely chopped fresh rosemary

I tablespoon extra-virgin olive oil

Jerusalem artichokes, also known as sunchokes, are neither from Jerusalem, nor botanically related to globe artichokes. Rather, these root vegetables are actually a relative of the sunflower and look like knobby potatoes. They have a subtle, nutty flavor and are perfectly suited to roasting, mashing, or in this case, slicing and baking into crispy chips. Not only are sunchokes delicious, they're also prebiotic powerhouses.

wild bonus: Jerusalem artichokes stimulate the growth of friendly bacteria such as bifidobacteria and help to suppress unfriendly bacteria in the gut.

Preheat the oven to 400°F. Line a large baking sheet with foil.

Gently scrub the sunchokes under cold running water. Cut them into ⅛-inch-thick slices with a sharp knife or a mandoline. Spread the slices on a paper towel and press down with another paper towel to remove as much moisture as possible.

With a mortar and pestle or in a small bowl using the back of a spoon, mash together the salt, lemon zest, and rosemary.

In a large bowl, toss together the sunchokes, salt/herb mixture, and olive oil until evenly coated. Arrange the sunchokes in a single layer on the prepared baking sheet. Bake for 15 minutes. Then, using tongs, give the sunchokes a toss and bake until golden and crisp, about another 15 minutes. Serve warm or at room temperature.

CATALAN GAZPACHO
Tomato · Cucumber · Almond

Serves 4

2 (1-inch thick) slices sprouted-grain bread (such as Ezekiel), crusts removed

2 small cucumbers, peeled, seeded, and chopped

2 pounds very ripe tomatoes, seeded and coarsely chopped

1 garlic clove, chopped

2 tablespoons blanched almonds

2 tablespoons sherry vinegar

1 tablespoon extra-virgin olive oil, plus more for drizzling

Celtic sea salt

Optional Garnishes:

Chopped toasted almonds

Chopped scallions

Chopped shallots

Sweet corn kernels

Crème fraîche

Have you made a chilled tomato soup when the tomatoes were in season and vine-ripened by the summer sun? Their perfumed sweetness makes any other tomato seem mealy and bland in comparison. So while this dish is really simple to make, the main ingredient can make or break it. Restaurants often try to disguise the quality of their tomatoes by adding sugar, but if your tomatoes are at their seasonal peak, you won't need the added sweetener. This Catalan version is pureed with almonds for a little more richness and body.

wild bonus: Almonds contain phytochemicals and fibers that help boost favorable strains of bacteria in the gut.

In a small bowl, submerge the bread in water and soak for at least 15 minutes. Drain, squeeze out the excess moisture, and place in a blender or food processor.

Add the cucumbers, tomatoes, garlic, almonds, vinegar, and olive oil to the bread. Add ½ cup water and puree until smooth, adding a bit more water if needed.

Strain the puree through a fine-mesh strainer into a bowl, using a back of a spoon to coax it through.

Season to taste with salt. (I don't use pepper in my gazpacho because I find it too overpowering.)

Chill the gazpacho in the refrigerator overnight or for at least a few hours. Spoon into a bowl, drizzle with olive oil, top with your garnishes of choice, and serve.

NOT-YOUR-TYPICAL GREEK SALAD

Cucumber · Walnuts · Rice · Cracked Pepper · Egg · Feta

Serves 2

2 cups cooked Arborio or long-grain rice

½ cup walnuts, crushed

Celtic sea salt and freshly ground black pepper

10 cherry or grape tomatoes, halved

1 medium cucumber, peeled and cut into bite-size pieces

1 small red onion, thinly sliced

2 tablespoons extra-virgin olive oil, plus more for drizzling

3 tablespoons crumbled feta cheese

2 Yiayia's Eggs Mati (page 96)

1 teaspoon dried oregano

I thought long and hard about how to put my own spin on this one. The classic version is absolutely perfect—especially when tomatoes are in season. But I wanted to do something with a little bit of a twist, creating a sort of salad parfait by layering rice with traditional Greek salad ingredients and topping them with a savory egg. This is hearty enough to be a main dish.

wild bonus: Increasing your fruit and vegetable intake is the best way to load up on antioxidants, which help your body detoxify.

In a medium bowl, combine the rice and walnuts. Season with salt and pepper to taste. Set aside.

In a large bowl, combine the tomatoes, cucumber, red onion, 2 tablespoons of the olive oil, and the feta and lightly toss the mixture together.

To serve, layer the bottom of each of two dinner plates with half of the rice mixture, using a spatula to pat it down. Scoop half of the salad ingredients onto each mound of rice and top each with one of Yiayia's Eggs. Season with the oregano and salt, cracked pepper, and a final drizzle of olive oil to taste.

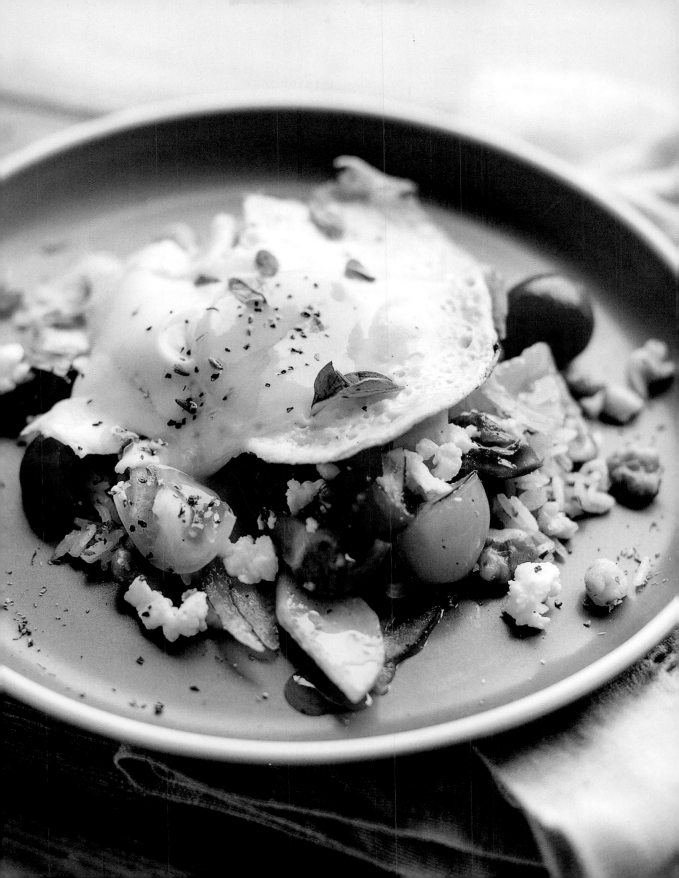

ST. BARTS-STYLE CHILLED PEA SOUP

Pea · Scallion · Creme

Serves 4

3 cups Roasted Vegetable Stock (page 174) or store-bought

24 ounces frozen peas or 4 cups fresh peas (from about 4 pounds in the pod)

5 scallions, white parts only, chopped

2 teaspoons Celtic sea salt, plus more to taste

I tablespoon extra-virgin olive oil

½ cup 2% Greek yogurt or ¼ cup crème fraîche

I teaspoon ground white pepper (optional)

St. Barts is a French colony in the Caribbean, and it inspired this brightly colored cold soup that's perfect for the warmer months. After all, France is known for its velvety chilled soups.

If you're not able to find fresh peas, you can always use frozen. And feel free to substitute crème fraîche for the yogurt; just reduce the amount to ¼ cup.

wild bonus: Peas are a healthy source of plant fiber, which helps keep the bacterial ecosystem in your gut thriving.

In a medium soup pot, bring the stock to a boil over high heat. Reduce the heat to a simmer and add the peas and scallion whites. Simmer for 5 minutes, taking care not to overcook the peas.

Remove from the heat and allow the soup to cool slightly. Using a food processor or immersion blender, puree the soup until smooth. Blend in the sea salt and olive oil. Pour the soup into a large bowl and stir in the yogurt.

Cover the bowl and refrigerate for at least 2 hours or preferably overnight until the soup is thoroughly chilled. Season with salt and white pepper, if desired, and serve.

GREEK WILD GREENS WITH OLIVE OIL AND LEMON

Sunchoke Chips · Olive Oil · Lemon

Serves 6

1 bunch Swiss chard, well washed and ribs removed

1 bunch mustard greens

2 tablespoons extra-virgin olive oil

Sunchoke Chips (optional; page 108), for serving

3 lemons, halved

Celtic sea salt

In Greece, *horta vrasta* (HOR-tah vrah-STAH) refers to collecting wild greens and braising them with a bit of lemon and olive oil. Once you've mastered the basic technique, try using whatever variety of greens you come across, either at the market or from your garden—from the tops of beets and turnips, to dandelion leaves, kale, escarole, or collards. There are wonderful Asian greens that can be used, too. Some people, like my grandmother, save and drink the cooking water to get every last bit of nutritional goodness. I remember taking a sip of this "green juice" when I was a little girl and thinking I'd never tasted anything so awful—it's not for the faint of heart! Luckily, you can reap this magical liquid's benefits without drinking it by making Yiayia's Horta Toner (page 206). You can also save the *horta* water and use it to make a simple vegetable stock.

wild bonus: Vegetables and salads made with wild greens have been a source of plant fibers and phytochemicals in the Mediterranean diet for centuries.

Bring a large pot of water to a boil.

Add the greens to the pot and boil until tender, about 20 minutes.

Drain the greens in a colander (set over a large bowl if keeping the cooking water for another use).

Allow the greens to cool. Serve chilled or at room temperature (depending on whether it's warm or cold outside) topped with the olive oil and Sunchoke Chips (if using). Set out lemon halves and sea salt so diners can season to their individual tastes.

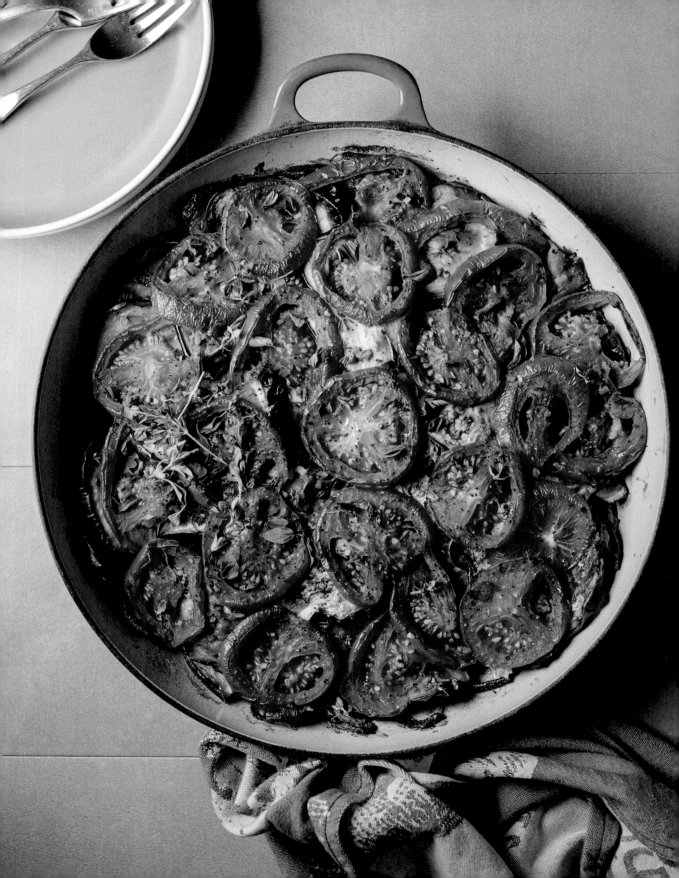

BRIAM

Potato · Vegetables · White Wine · Olive Oil

Serves 8

¾ cup extra-virgin olive oil, plus more for baking and serving

3 large russet potatoes, scrubbed and cut into ½-inch-thick slices

5 medium yellow potatoes, scrubbed and cut into ½-inch-thick slices

I large eggplant, cut into ½-inch-thick slices

5 zucchini, cut into ½-inch-thick slices

2 teaspoons Celtic sea salt

½ cup dry white wine

I cup tomato paste

I teaspoon freshly ground black pepper

2 tablespoons dried oregano

10 cherry tomatoes, halved

I medium onion, diced

5 garlic cloves, minced

4 large tomatoes, cut into ¼-inch-thick slices

2 tablespoons chopped fresh flat-leaf parsley

If you really want to understand exactly how generously olive oil is used in Greek cuisine, then you need to try this braised vegetable dish—just don't freak out when you see the quantity of EVOO called for. It's a lot, but a Greek cook would probably use twice as much! The idea is to flavor the vegetables with the natural nutty-fruit flavor of the oil while making the vegetables super soft and aromatic. Similar versions can be found in the cooking of Italy (*verdure brasate*), France (ratatouille), and Spain (*estofado de verduras*). I make this dish with two different types of potato—white russet and yellow (unlike traditional versions, I leave mine unpeeled to reap all that great fiber)—along with eggplant, zucchini, tomatoes, onion, and garlic, although you could swap in any vegetables you like. Choose a healthy-looking eggplant that's firm to the touch, and the thickest zucchini you can find, and keep everything in a circular pattern when layering the vegetables for the prettiest presentation. This dish is best cooked in a Dutch oven or earthenware baking dish that can comfortably hold a layer of vegetables about 4 inches deep. For the best flavor, let the dish rest for a few hours. The juices released by the vegetables will reabsorb and make this dish super tasty. I always felt that aside from the quality of vegetables and olive oil (which is really important), allowing the dish to "sit" was one of the secrets to making a star-worthy *briam*.

wild bonus: This dish pairs well with animal-based proteins, helping you achieve the perfect plant fiber-to-protein ratio.

Preheat the oven to 400°F. Lightly oil two large baking sheets with olive oil.

Spread the sliced potatoes, eggplant, and zucchini on the sheets in a single layer. You may need to do this in batches if they don't

(recipe continues)

all fit in a single layer in two pans. Drizzle the vegetables with some olive oil and sprinkle with 1 teaspoon of the salt. Roast the vegetables for 20 minutes, turning once at the halfway point. Take the vegetables out, but leave the oven on.

Meanwhile, in a medium bowl, mix together the ¾ cup olive oil, wine, tomato paste, remaining 1 teaspoon salt, and the pepper.

Oil the bottom and sides of a Dutch oven or deep ovenproof pan. Working in a circular pattern, use half of the potatoes to line the bottom of the pan. Scatter a few pinches of oregano over the potatoes and continue layering with the eggplant, zucchini, cherry tomatoes, onion, garlic, the remaining potatoes, and the sliced tomatoes, adding a sprinkle of oregano to each layer.

Drizzle the olive oil/wine/tomato mixture over the top of the vegetables. Sprinkle a bit of oregano over the top. Bake until the potatoes on top are soft, about 30 minutes.

Allow the dish to cool completely before serving. Garnish with parsley before serving.

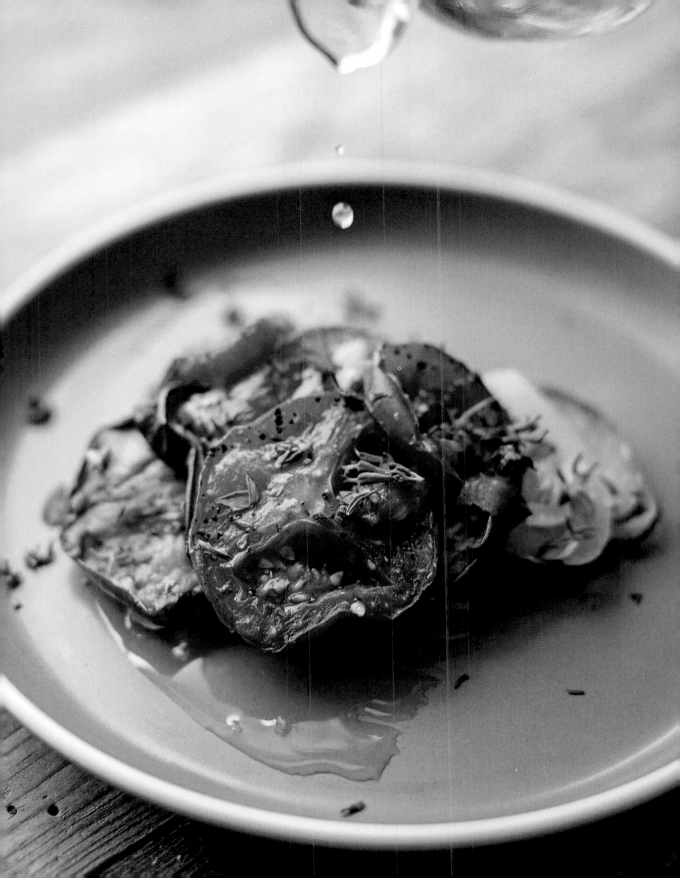

SPINACH PIE WITH SPROUTED WHEAT CRUST

Sprouted Wheat · Feta · Paprika · Ricotta

Serves 6 to 8

This recipe is an updated rendition of the classic spanakopita, a Greek spinach pie usually made with flaky phyllo dough. This version instead uses a dough made from sprouted-wheat flour and olive oil, with just a bit of butter incorporated into the final product. I have also added ricotta to make the filling nice and creamy.

wild bonus: Sprouted-wheat flour is generally considered superior to processed flours because the wheat is soaked and sprouted before it is milled into flour, which helps increase its nutritional value. Both King Arthur and Arrowhead Mills offer sprouted-wheat flours that are widely available.

For the Crust:

2 cups sprouted-wheat flour, plus more for dusting

1 teaspoon fine Celtic sea salt

1 teaspoon dried thyme

⅓ cup extra-virgin olive oil, plus more for the pan

⅔ cup cold water

For the Filling:

2 tablespoons extra-virgin olive oil

2 pounds spinach, washed, dried, thick stems discarded, and coarsely chopped

1 bunch scallions (about 3 ounces), white and light green parts only, finely chopped

1 medium onion, chopped

2 garlic cloves, minced

8 ounces crumbled feta cheese

8 ounces whole-milk ricotta cheese

To make the crust: In a medium bowl, combine the flour, salt, and thyme. Add the oil and mix it in with your fingers until the oil is distributed evenly. It should have the consistency of coarse cornmeal. Mix in the water until absorbed, then knead the mixture lightly by hand until the dough comes together into a ball. Divide the dough into two balls. Wrap one ball in plastic and place it in the fridge to rest.

Turn out the other ball of dough onto a lightly floured surface. Sprinkle a little flour on the dough and a rolling pin, and roll the dough out into a round large enough to fit a 9-inch pie pan, turning the dough slightly every time you roll it. Dust the dough with flour to keep it from becoming sticky. Avoid overworking it.

Lightly grease the 9-inch pie pan with olive oil. Transfer the dough to the pan and trim the excess. Let it rest in the fridge for 25 minutes while you prepare the filling.

2 tablespoons finely grated Greek kefalotyri cheese or Parmigiano-Reggiano

3 eggs, beaten

⅓ cup finely chopped fresh dill

⅓ cup finely chopped fresh flat-leaf parsley

½ teaspoon freshly ground black pepper

¼ teaspoon freshly grated nutmeg

½ teaspoon Celtic sea salt, or to taste

1 tablespoon unsalted butter, melted

1 teaspoon paprika (optional)

To make the filling: In a large skillet, heat 1 tablespoon of the oil over medium-high heat. Add the spinach a few handfuls at a time, tossing the spinach with tongs and adding more as each batch begins to wilt. Cook until all the spinach is wilted. Using a slotted spoon or spatula, transfer the spinach to a colander or large plate lined with paper towels to capture any excess water and oil. Once the spinach is cool enough to touch, use your hands to wring out as much of the remaining liquid as possible.

Wipe the pan dry and heat the remaining tablespoon of oil over medium heat. Add the scallions and onion and cook until softened, about 5 minutes. Stir in the garlic and cook for 1 additional minute. Stir the spinach into the onion mixture, then remove from the heat. Allow the spinach and onion mixture to cool for a few minutes. Stir in the feta, ricotta, kefalotyri, eggs, dill, parsley, pepper, nutmeg, and salt until they're thoroughly combined.

When you're ready to assemble the pie, preheat the oven to 400°F.

Remove the remaining ball of dough from the fridge and roll it out to a 14-inch round. Spread the spinach filling into the prepared crust in the pan. Cover the filling with the top crust and, using your fingers, pinch the top and bottom crusts' edges together, trimming as needed. Brush the top with the melted butter and dust it with the paprika (if using).

Bake the pie until the crust is nicely browned, about 45 minutes. Transfer to a wire rack to cool completely before serving.

LEGUMES, SEEDS, AND GRAINS

——

Although I do not recommend eating heavy portions of grains, you can enjoy them in moderation, as a satisfying supplement to the main meal. Rice and pasta are staples for most Mediterranean cultures, and a way to extend more costly ingredients like seafood, as in my Paella (page 133). Sprouted grains bring healthy nutrients as well as toothsome bite to pizza crusts and tortillas, proving there is a place for everything on the Wild Mediterranean table. Legumes, on the other hand, are a wonderful source of protein (as are seeds), and they also improve the quality of the field in which they are grown. Many of these legumes end up in the region's side dishes, often braised in homemade stock coupled with a local vegetable or two, like the Fava recipe on page 125.

FOUR COUNTRIES, FOUR WAYS: **BEANS**

Beans are loaded with protein and plant fiber (the kind that's so great at giving your digestive system a good scrub), but they're also a great canvas for all kinds of ingredients and flavors. With a few simple swaps you can change from Greek-style beans with tomatoes, herbs, and feta to Spanish-style accented with sausage, sun-dried tomato, and parsley.

Buy from a farmers' market or store with a high turnover, as old beans can take as much as three times longer than fresher ones to soften when cooking. (There's also no shame in using canned beans. Just make sure the can is BPA-free.) If you avoid beans because of their reputed side effects, I recommend soaking your beans with a small piece of seaweed. Sea vegetables such as kelp or kombu help break down the enzymes that can make beans hard to digest and, in turn, lead to gas.

wild bonus: Beans help produce short-chain fatty acids (SCFAs), which help intestinal flora flourish in a healthy, balanced way.

COOKING DRIED BEANS

I pound dried beans	I teaspoon Celtic sea salt
I piece of kombu (about 3 inches)	I bay leaf

Put the beans in a medium pot and add enough cold water to cover by at least 3 inches. Add the kombu and soak the beans overnight. Or do a "rapid soak" by bringing the beans to a boil and cooking for 2 minutes. Remove the pot from the heat, cover, and let sit for 1 hour.

Drain the beans, discarding the kombu, and return them to the pot. Cover with fresh cold water and bring to a boil. Skim any scum that rises to the surface. Add the salt and bay leaf, reduce to a gentle simmer, and cover. After about 45 minutes, remove the lid and skim off any foam. Test the beans to see if they've softened. If not, cook until a sampling of a few beans assures they're uniformly tender, another 10 minutes or so.

Drain the beans in a sieve set over a large bowl. Reserve the cooking liquid separately.

MAKING BAKED BEANS

Preheat the oven to 350°F.

In a medium soup pot or Dutch oven, cook the sauté ingredients (see the variations that follow) over medium heat until softened, 2 to 3 minutes.

(recipe continues)

Stir in the cooked beans, cover, and transfer the pot to the oven. Bake until the vegetables have all cooked through and the mixture is fragrant, about 30 minutes.

To serve, season the beans with salt, pepper, and extra-virgin olive oil. Garnish with any additional toppings.

GREEK-STYLE BAKED BEANS
Tomatoes · Dill · Feta

Serves 6

For the Beans:

I pound dried butter beans, cooked

For the Sauté:

I tablespoon unsalted butter

I large Spanish onion, finely chopped

2 large carrots, finely chopped

3 celery stalks, finely chopped

2 garlic cloves, minced

For Baking:

I pound tomatoes, peeled and finely chopped, or I can (14 ounces) crushed tomatoes

¼ cup extra-virgin olive oil

I tablespoon tomato paste

¼ cup chopped fresh dill

I teaspoon sugar

I teaspoon dried oregano

Pinch of ground cinnamon

Freshly cracked black pepper, to taste

For Serving:

Celtic sea salt and freshly ground black pepper

Extra-virgin olive oil

½ cup crumbled feta cheese, for topping

Fresh flat-leaf parsley, chopped, for topping

SPANISH-STYLE BAKED BEANS
Sausage · Sun-Dried Tomato · Parsley

Serves 4 to 6

To give this a stew-like consistency, add 4 cups chicken, beef, or vegetable stock before baking.

For the Beans:

I pound dried cannellini beans, cooked

For the Sauté:

I tablespoon unsalted butter

2 fully cooked organic turkey or chicken sausages, cut into bite-size pieces

I medium onion, diced

2 garlic cloves, minced

For Baking:

I cup diced sun-dried tomatoes

6 cups shredded baby spinach leaves (or other greens such as collards, kale, or dandelion)

I tablespoon olive oil

½ cup chopped fresh flat-leaf parsley

I teaspoon sugar

I teaspoon dried oregano

Freshly cracked black pepper, to taste

For Serving:

Celtic sea salt and freshly ground black pepper

Extra-virgin olive oil

FRENCH-STYLE BAKED BEANS

Shallots · Thyme · Mushroom

Serves 4 to 6

For the Beans:

1 pound dried cannellini beans, cooked

For the Sauté:

1 tablespoon unsalted butter

1 large shallot, thinly sliced

6 cremini mushrooms, trimmed and chopped

1 garlic clove, thinly sliced

For Baking:

½ cup dry white wine

2 tablespoons extra-virgin olive oil

1 teaspoon granulated sugar

1 teaspoon fresh thyme

For Serving:

Extra-virgin olive oil

Celtic sea salt and ground black pepper

Chopped fresh flat-leaf parsley, for topping

ITALIAN-STYLE BEAN SALAD

Frisée · Tuna · Vinaigrette

Serves 6

This variation is slightly different in that it's not baked; it's more of a salad that is served at room temperature.

1 head frisée, cored and leaves torn into bite-size pieces

Extra-virgin olive oil

Celtic sea salt and freshly ground black pepper

1 pound dried cannellini beans or other small white bean, cooked

2 celery stalks, thinly sliced

2 (6-ounce) cans tuna, packed in water or oil, drained

3 to 4 tablespoons Wild Vinaigrette (page 173)

½ cup chopped fresh flat-leaf parsley

Place the frisée in a large bowl. Drizzle with olive oil and season with salt and pepper to taste, then toss well to coat. Set aside.

In another large bowl, combine the cooked beans and celery. Season with salt and pepper.

Spread the dressed frisée on a large serving platter. Layer the beans on top of the greens and top with the tuna. Drizzle the vinaigrette over all and garnish with the parsley.

Note: Water-packed tuna will have a milder flavor, while oil-packed is richer; my favorite brand is Wild Planet.

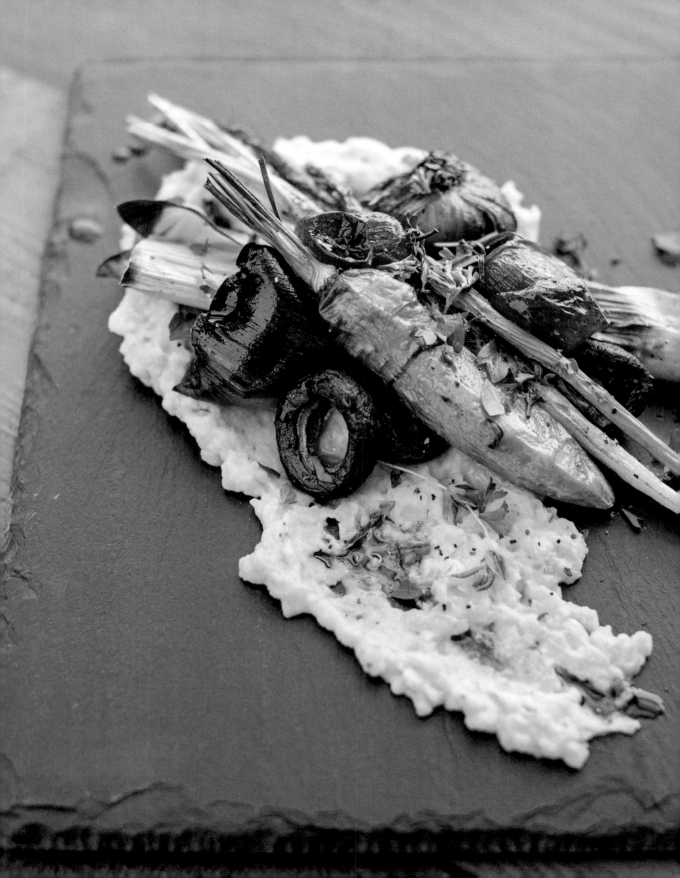

FAVA WITH ROASTED VEGETABLES

Olive Oil · Sea Salt · Yellow Split Peas

Serves 4 to 6

⅓ cup, plus 3 tablespoons extra-virgin olive oil, plus more for drizzling

3 red onions, roughly chopped (1 tablespoon set aside for garnish)

2 garlic cloves, chopped

2 cups yellow split peas, rinsed well

1 tablespoon fresh lemon juice

4 shallots, peeled and halved

15 asparagus stalks, trimmed

10 small tomatoes, cored

10 white or cremini mushrooms, trimmed

5 carrots, peeled

2 leeks, white and light green parts only, well washed and patted dry

1 tablespoon dried thyme

Celtic sea salt and freshly ground black pepper

Fava (not to be confused with fava beans) is a puree of cooked yellow split peas, flavored with onion and olive oil. The smokiness of the peas plays against the caramelized sweetness of the vegetables beautifully. It's ultrasimple, but there's a secret: The type of olive oil you use can make or break this dish. Using a high-quality extra-virgin olive oil is a must. Its acidity and fruity flavor perfectly balance the dish. Feel free to play around with dried and fresh herbs for seasoning.

wild bonus: Yellow split peas contain a type of fiber known as resistant starch that's particularly beneficial for intestinal microbiota.

In a large pot, heat 1 tablespoon of the olive oil over medium-high heat. Add the onions and garlic and sauté until softened, about 3 minutes. Add the yellow split peas and stir well. Pour in enough water to cover the peas by 1 inch (about 6 cups). Reduce the heat, cover, and simmer until the peas have begun to break apart, about 30 minutes. Now and then use a spoon to skim off any white foam that rises to the surface.

Drain the peas, then transfer them to a blender or food processor. Add the lemon juice and pulse a few times, then continue to pulse as you add the remaining ⅓ cup olive oil. Season with salt and pepper. I prefer a slightly grainy consistency, but you can make it as chunky or smooth as you like. Transfer to a bowl, cover, and refrigerate to let the flavors meld.

Preheat the oven to 450°F.

(recipe continues)

On a large baking sheet, combine the shallots, asparagus, tomatoes, mushrooms, carrots, and leeks. Toss with about 2 tablespoons of the olive oil, the thyme, and a pinch each of salt and pepper. Roast until all the vegetables are tender and beginning to caramelize, 15 to 20 minutes, turning once or twice to ensure they cook evenly.

Serve the puree drizzled with some extra-virgin olive oil and sprinkled with the reserved chopped onions. Top with the roasted vegetables and another drizzle of oil.

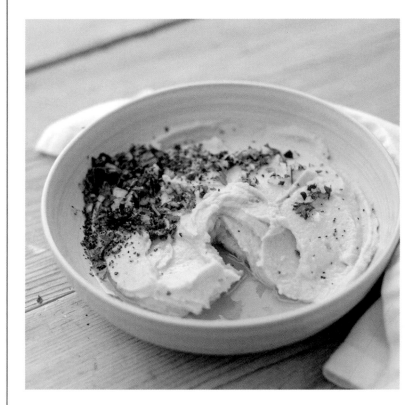

ROASTED SQUASH SEEDS WITH SEA SALT

Olive Oil · Salt · Spice

Makes about 1 cup

Seeds from I butternut
squash

I to 2 tablespoons
olive oil

Fine Celtic sea salt

Villagers would never throw away the protein-packed seeds of
a squash. In modern times, it's still worth taking an extra step to
make a snack or salad topper that's high in protein, lipids, and fiber.
It's best to roast the seeds *after* the squash (instead of together)
because they need to roast at a lower temperature in order not to
burn. This also works for seeds from any winter squash, including
pumpkins of course. Once you've got the technique down, try adding
½ teaspoon of spices such as paprika, garlic, or chili powder for
amped-up flavor.

wild bonus: This recipe is high in plant-based protein, which is an
essential ingredient for diversifying the microbiome.

Preheat the oven to 275°F. Line a large baking sheet with foil or
parchment paper.

Rinse the seeds with water and rub them with your fingertips to
remove any stringy leftover bits of pulp. Pat them dry and put
them in a small bowl. Toss the seeds with enough olive oil just
to coat and a pinch of sea salt. Spread them evenly on the lined
baking sheet.

Bake until the seeds start to pop, about 15 minutes. Let the seeds
cool on the baking sheet. Store in an airtight container at room
temperature for up to 1 week.

MYCONIAN-INSPIRED BLACK-EYED PEAS

Grilled Peaches • Mint • Parmigiano-Reggiano

Serves 4 to 6

2 peaches

½ cup extra-virgin olive oil

Celtic sea salt

1 can (14 ounces) black-eyed peas, drained

20 fresh mint leaves (¼ cup packed)

¼ cup freshly grated Parmigiano-Reggiano cheese

Freshly ground black pepper

Nikolas Taverna in Mykonos serves incredibly delicious black-eyed peas, which inspired this dish. Combined with the smoky-sweet grilled peaches, bright mint, and salty Parmigiano, humble black-eyed peas become downright crave-worthy. If it's not barbecue season, you can "grill" the peaches—or any other stone fruit—in a cast-iron grill pan. Also, I find that using a little more olive oil than most calorie-conservative folks might like really enlivens this dish. There's no need to fear healthy fats!

wild bonus: Black-eyed peas contain a healthy dose of folate, which is a natural mood booster.

Cut the peaches along the seam all the way around and twist the halves off the pit. Brush the cut sides with a bit of the olive oil and sprinkle with a pinch of salt.

Lay the peaches cut-side down on a grill or grill pan over high heat. Cook until grill marks form, about 3 minutes. Brush the skin side with a bit more olive oil, flip, and grill for another 3 minutes. When the peaches are cool enough to handle, thinly slice them.

Combine the sliced grilled peaches with the black-eyed peas and mint leaves, drizzle with olive oil, and top with Parmigiano plus a bit of salt and pepper.

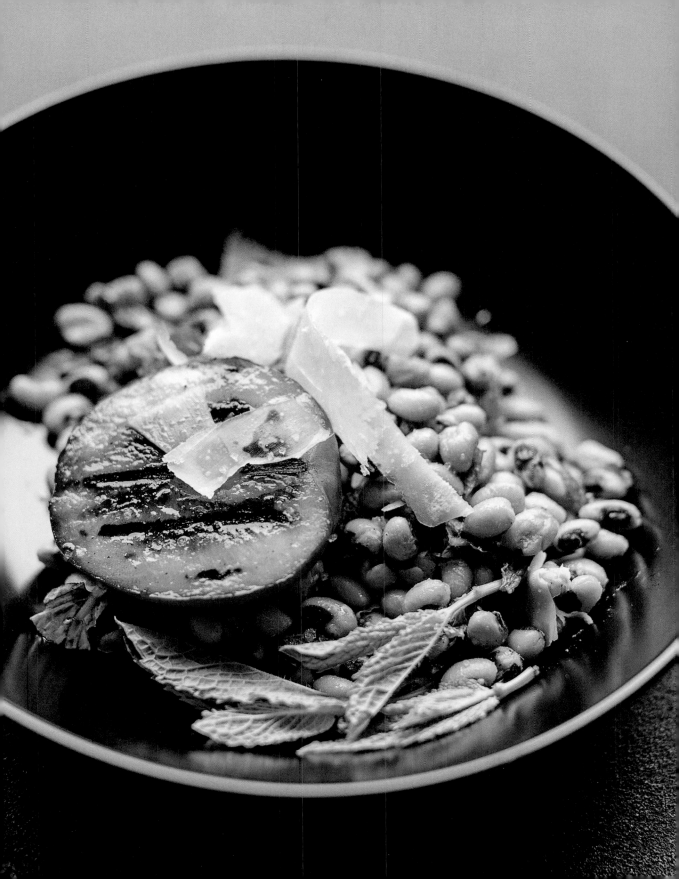

RIGATONI WITH BUTTERNUT SQUASH AND BASIL

Basil · Butternut Squash · Sheep's Cheese

Serves 6

I medium butternut squash (I to 1½ pounds)

4 tablespoons extra-virgin olive oil, plus more for serving

I tablespoon dried thyme

Celtic sea salt

16 ounces rigatoni

I teaspoon freshly ground black pepper

I tablespoon chopped fresh basil, plus more for garnish

⅔ cup Roasted Vegetable Stock (page 174) or store-bought

Pecorino and Parmigiano-Reggiano cheese, for serving

Although processed wheat products like pasta are not at the top of my recommended list, once you have re-wilded your gut, it's okay to enjoy foods you really miss on the rare occasion. For those times I wanted to create a classic Italian pasta dish that wasn't based on tomato sauce, because canned tomatoes can be problematic for some. The result is an easy-to-prepare marinara alternative that works just as well for pasta as it does for lasagna and pizza. It takes less time than you might think to cut up a squash, plus you can roast the seeds (page 127) and sprinkle them on your favorite salad with Wild Vinaigrette (page 173). However, starting with precut fresh or frozen squash is fine, too.

I should also note that I've made this recipe with brown rice and quinoa fusilli as well as traditional pasta like the rigatoni in this recipe. Organic pasta would be the best choice and it has become widely available. If gluten-free pasta if desired, avoid the corn-based versions because they really don't hold together well after cooking. Opt for a brown rice version instead.

wild bonus: Butternut squash contains beta-carotene, a contributor to mucosal homeostasis in the gut.

Preheat the oven to 350°F.

Halve the butternut squash lengthwise and use a spoon to scoop out the seeds, reserving them to roast, if desired. Place both halves, cut-side up, on a baking sheet. Brush the flesh with 1 tablespoon of the olive oil and season with the thyme and salt to taste. Bake until the squash is fork-tender, about 25 minutes. Then remove from the oven and allow it to cool.

Meanwhile, bring a pot of water to a boil. Add the rigatoni with a generous amount of salt and cook according to package instructions until al dente. Drain.

Once the squash is cool enough to handle, scoop the flesh into a large bowl, discarding the skin. Mash the squash with a fork, then add the remaining 3 tablespoons olive oil, 2 teaspoons salt, the pepper, basil, and vegetable stock.

Gently toss the squash mixture with the cooked pasta and serve with torn fresh basil leaves, a drizzle of olive oil, a sprinkle of sea salt, and a fresh grating of cheese.

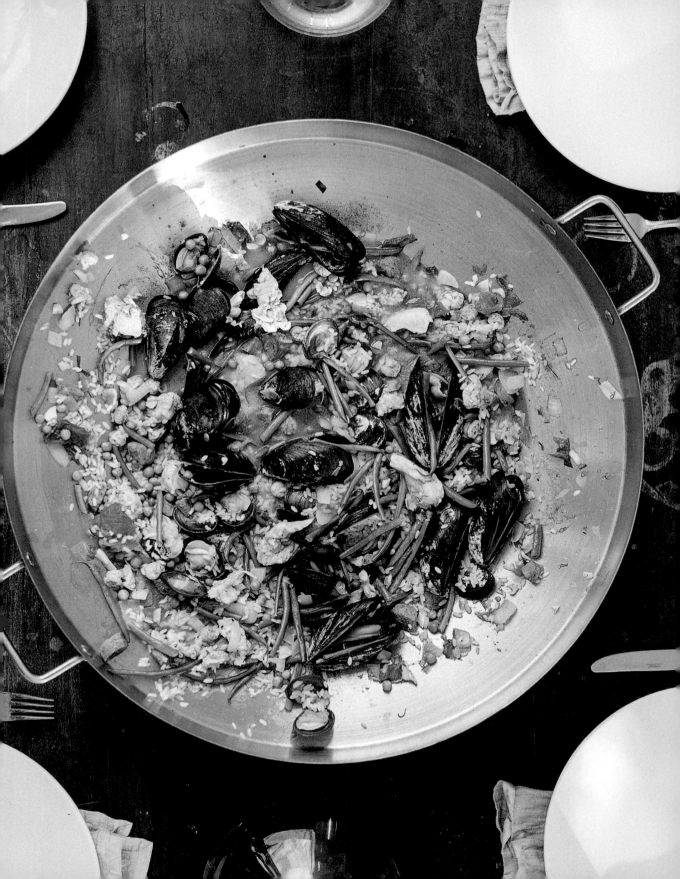

JACKSON POLLOCK'S PAELLA

Saffron Rice · Orange Zest · Fish

Serves 6

2 tablespoons extra-virgin olive oil

8 ounces nitrate-free chicken sausage without pork casings (I like Applegate), cut in bite-size pieces

8 boneless, skinless chicken thighs, chopped into bite-size pieces

4 garlic cloves, minced

I large yellow onion, diced

2 large tomatoes, seeded and chopped

6 cups Fish Stock (page 175) or store-bought

2 cups bomba or Arborio rice

1½ teaspoons saffron threads

I teaspoon dried thyme

Celtic sea salt and freshly ground black pepper

I pound medium shrimp, peeled and deveined

I pound mussels, bearded and scrubbed

I named this recipe after the artist Jackson Pollock because paella—a traditional Spanish dish of vibrant saffron-yellow rice studded with a mix of meats and seafood plus a medley of aromatics and vegetables—reminds me of his art. I know it looks like there's a lot to do here, but it's really just a one-pot casserole.

This recipe calls for a 12- or 15-inch paella pan, but if you don't have one, a 12-inch or larger shallow skillet will work. Also, if you can find Spanish bomba rice, I highly recommend you use it, as it can absorb almost twice as much liquid as other varieties without getting mushy. If not, Arborio is a great alternative.

wild bonus: Fish is a rich source of iodine and magnesium, two very important minerals for maintaining a healthy gut.

Heat a large paella pan or skillet over medium-high heat or on a hot grill. Add the oil and sauté the sausage until cooked through, 8 to 12 minutes. Remove the sausage from the pan and drain off all but about ¼ cup of fat. Add the chicken to the pan and cook, turning occasionally, until cooked through, about 15 minutes. Remove the chicken from the pan and set aside.

Combine the garlic, onion, and tomatoes in the pan and cook until softened, about 3 minutes. Add the fish stock, return the sausage and chicken to the pan, and cook over medium heat for 10 minutes.

Add the rice and cook, stirring, for about 3 minutes. Add the saffron, thyme, several gratings of black pepper, and 3 pinches of salt. Stir as the mixture comes back to a boil.

(recipe continues)

1½ cups green beans (preferably haricots vert), trimmed and halved

2 cups frozen peas

2 to 3 lemons, cut into wedges

Cover the pan loosely with foil and continue to cook until the rice is tender, about 25 minutes. Do not stir during that time—the steam will help the rice cook evenly. If excess liquid remains, remove the foil and let the mixture continue to cook until the liquid has been fully absorbed.

Add the shrimp, mussels, and green beans to the rice mixture. Toss the peas on top. Cover again until the seafood cooks through, about 10 minutes. Remove the pot from the heat and let it stand, covered, for a couple of minutes before serving. Discard any mussels that have not opened. Serve with the lemon wedges.

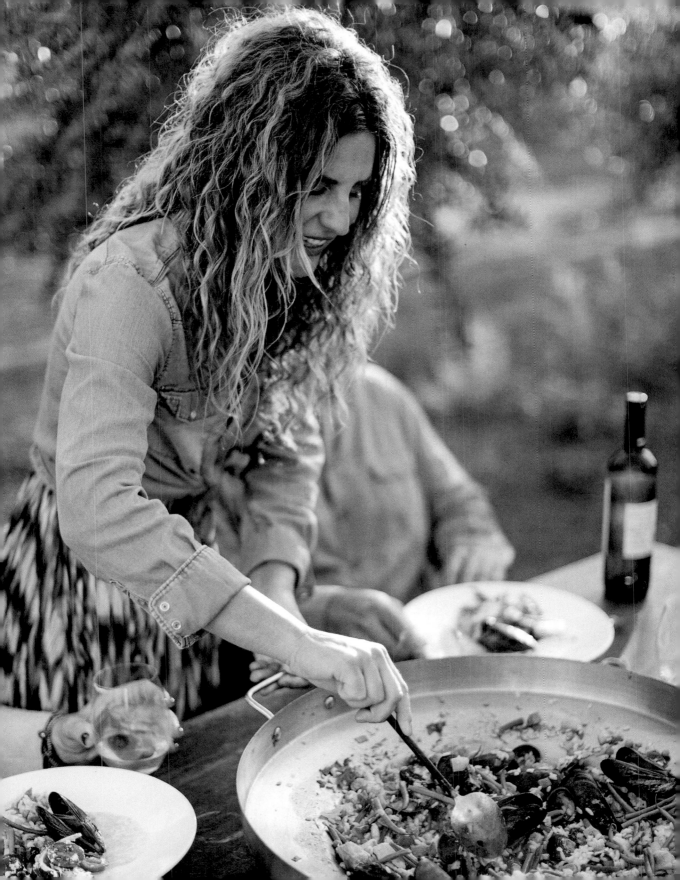

RISOTTO CLASSICO

Mascarpone · Shallot · Tangerine

Serves 4

1 unwaxed tangerine

1 tablespoon unsalted butter

3 tablespoons extra-virgin olive oil

1 shallot, thinly sliced

1½ cups Arborio rice

1 cup dry white wine

4 cups Mineral-Rich Bone Broth (page 176) or store-bought low-sodium chicken stock, heated to a simmer

3 tablespoons mascarpone

3 tablespoons grated Parmesan cheese

Celtic sea salt and freshly ground black pepper

Rich, decadent risotto is hard to beat for a special meal. The one cardinal rule for making this dish: Don't rush it. Be sure the shallots are translucent before you begin adding the rice, and that the rice is a milky-white color before adding the liquid. Toasting the rice in the fats without any liquid is a key step as it helps determine the final texture of the rice. Be sure to use warm stock; adding cold stock to the hot rice will cook the outside of the rice, but not the inside, resulting in a hard, unpleasant texture.

wild bonus: Although this dish is starch heavy, it includes the mineral-boosting properties of the broth.

Grate the zest of the tangerine (taking care not to include any of the bitter white pith) and then juice the tangerine. Set aside.

In a heavy saucepan, melt the butter into the olive oil over medium heat. Add the shallot and cook until translucent, about 3 minutes. Add the rice, stirring to coat with the oil. Cook until the rice is hot and pearly white but not brown, about 4 minutes. Stir in the wine and let it reduce by half, about 2 minutes. Add one ladle (about ½ cup) of warm broth and stir until it's incorporated into the rice.

Continue this process, stirring and adding about ½ cup of broth at a time, for about 15 minutes, and then taste a grain of rice. It should have a slight resistance when chewed. If it seems too hard, add ¼ cup more broth and continue cooking for another few minutes until the broth has been absorbed.

Remove the pot from the heat and let it sit for about 2 minutes. Stir in the mascarpone, Parmesan, and tangerine zest. Season to taste with salt and pepper.

PIZZA À LA STELLA

Basil · Mozzarella · Tomato · Black Olives

Serves 1

2 tablespoons tomato paste

2 teaspoons dried oregano

Fine Celtic sea salt

1 (regular size) sprouted-grain tortilla (such as Food For Life Ezekiel)

½ cup shredded part-skim mozzarella cheese

1 small tomato, thinly sliced and seeded

8 small black olives, pitted and diced

3 to 4 fresh basil leaves, torn

I couldn't dream of living without pizza, but like a lot of us, I suffer from digestive issues when I gobble up a greasy superprocessed slice. When I discovered that a sprouted-wheat tortilla makes an ideal base for a pizza, it made my day! I promise you won't miss the traditional processed crust in this easy-to-prepare version that sings with the flavors of the Mediterranean in every tasty bite. I use black olives most of the time, but feel free to use any other olive you like.

wild bonus: This "pizza" uses a tortilla made with sprouted-wheat flour, which is much more nutrient-rich than processed flours.

Preheat the oven to 350°F. Lightly oil a pizza stone or a heavy baking sheet and place in the oven to heat.

In a small bowl, stir together the tomato paste, 1 tablespoon water, 1 teaspoon of the oregano, and a pinch of salt. Add more water if necessary to create a smooth paste.

Place the tortilla on a flat work surface and spread the tomato mixture evenly over it. Sprinkle half the mozzarella cheese on top and arrange the tomato slices over the cheese. Season with a pinch of salt. Scatter the olives evenly over the top, along with the remaining mozzarella and the basil leaves.

Bake on the stone or baking sheet until the edges are crisp and the cheese has melted, about 15 minutes. Just before serving, sprinkle with the remaining 1 teaspoon oregano.

MAINS FROM
THE LAND

══

Villagers are true masters when it comes to working the land and reaping all its bounty, and they tend their animals with equal care, making sure they get all the sun and fresh feed they need to flourish. When it comes time to harvest those animals, they do so with respect. From meaty shanks to marrow for bone broth, it is the village way to make sure no part goes to waste.

CALIFORNIA-STYLE HOMEMADE GYRO WITH SPROUTED TORTILLA AND TZATZIKI

Meat · Garlic · Tomato · Onion

Serves 4 to 6

1 medium yellow onion

2 pounds lean ground lamb, chicken, or beef (or a mix of equal parts lamb and beef)

2 garlic cloves, minced

2 teaspoons dried oregano

1 teaspoon dried parsley

2 teaspoons Celtic sea salt

2 teaspoons onion powder

1 teaspoon garlic powder

1 teaspoon freshly ground black pepper

1 teaspoon ground cinnamon

½ teaspoon grated nutmeg

Sprouted-grain tortillas, regular size (such as Food For Life Ezekiel), lightly toasted, for serving

1 medium tomato, sliced, for serving

1 medium cucumber, sliced, for serving

Mom's Secret Tzatziki (page 177)

I'm not a fan of what has become of the gyro. Nowadays they're stuffed with heavily processed ingredients that include a host of binders and fillers, exactly the stuff I advise you to stay away from. Luckily, it's easy to make your own delicious (and healthy) version. Traditionally, you'd slowly roast a ton of meat on a spit, but roasting the meat in a loaf pan is so much easier. Then all you have to do is heat up a sprouted tortilla so it's warm and firm before wrapping it into a pita-style gyro. This is a favorite dish of all my Greek friends who love gyro but want the healthy "California" version.

Using a food processor, finely grate the onion. Add the meat, garlic, oregano, parsley, salt, onion powder, garlic powder, pepper, cinnamon, and nutmeg to the processor and pulse until the meat is sticky to the touch. Wrap the meat in plastic and transfer it to a 9 × 5-inch loaf pan. Refrigerate for a few hours or overnight.

Preheat the oven to 350°F.

Remove the meat from the plastic wrap and press it firmly into the loaf pan. Place the pan in a larger roasting pan and fill that with enough warm water to reach halfway up the sides of the loaf pan. Bake the meatloaf until an instant-read thermometer registers 170°F, about 30 minutes. Remove the loaf from the oven and allow it to rest for 10 to 15 minutes before slicing it lengthwise into 1-inch gyro strips.

Serve the gyro on the toasted tortillas with tomatoes, cucumbers, and tzatziki.

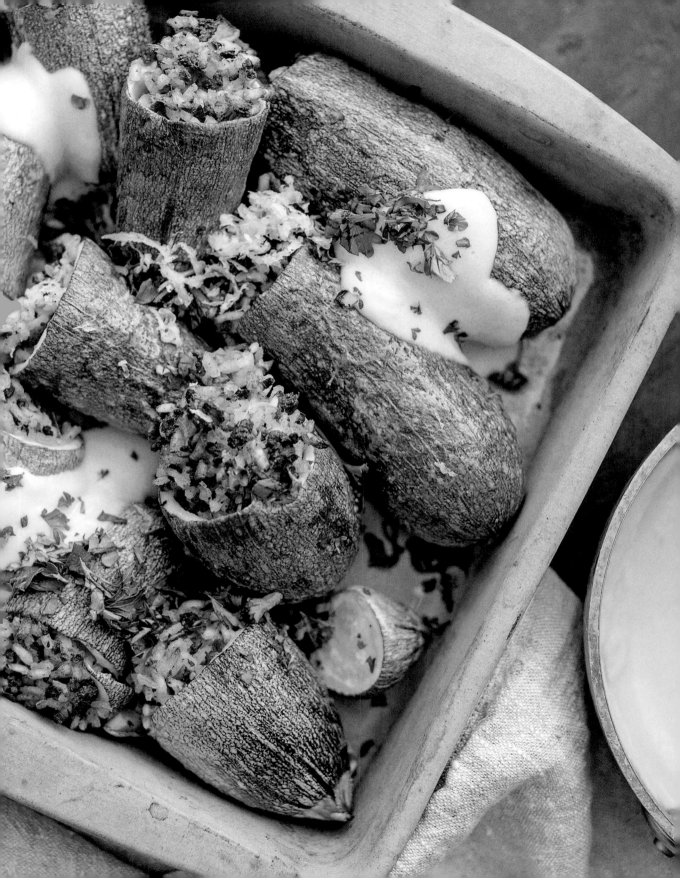

FROM-THE-VILLAGE STUFFED ZUCCHINI

Zucchini · Meat · Lemon Zest · Dill

Serves 4

For the Zucchini:

4 large zucchini, halved crosswise

2 teaspoons unsalted butter

I small yellow onion, chopped (about ¾ cup)

Celtic sea salt

3 garlic cloves, minced

½ pound ground beef, turkey, or lamb

1¾ cups Mineral-Rich Bone Broth (page 176) or store-bought low-sodium chicken stock

¾ cup Arborio or long-grain rice

2 tablespoons chopped fresh dill

¼ cup chopped fresh flat-leaf parsley

2 teaspoons chopped fresh mint

2 teaspoons grated lemon zest

¼ teaspoon freshly ground black pepper

I egg white (save the yolk for the sauce)

This classic Greek summer dish is typically made with a light-skinned summer squash known as marrow vegetable, but zucchini or any other summer squash make a perfect substitute. The vegetables are hollowed out and then stuffed with meat and herbs, so select the thickest zucchini or squash you can find. A zesty, creamy avgolemono sauce balances the savory meat stuffing. This dish is all about the sauce, so I make sure to follow the French way and add some extra fat by way of EVOO and an extra egg yolk.

You can prep the stuffed zucchini or squash a day early, then cover and refrigerate until you're ready to cook. And while this dish is traditionally made with beef or lamb, you can also use turkey, or a blend of meats, depending on your preference. When you make this you've got the perfect 3:1 veg-to-protein ratio in the bag!

To prepare the zucchini: Use a corer, melon baller, or sharp spoon to hollow out the zucchini halves. The remaining walls of the vegetable should be thin, yet sturdy enough to hold the meat stuffing. Mince the scooped-out zucchini pulp and set it aside.

In a large skillet, melt the butter over medium heat. Add the onion and sauté, adding a pinch of salt to help the onions soften. Cook until tender, 3 to 4 minutes. Add the garlic and cook for another minute. Transfer the vegetables to a bowl and set aside.

Increase the heat under the pan to medium-high, add the ground meat, and cook until browned, 8 to 10 minutes. Carefully drain off the excess fat, then return the onion-garlic mixture to the pan along with 1 cup of the broth, the rice, dill, parsley, mint, lemon

(recipe continues)

For the Avgolemono Sauce:

3 egg yolks

Juice of 1 lemon

½ cup low-sodium chicken broth, warmed

1 tablespoon extra-virgin olive oil

Celtic sea salt

2 ounces feta cheese, crumbled, for garnish (optional)

zest, pepper, and the minced zucchini pulp. Reduce the heat and simmer until the rice is cooked, about 20 minutes.

Transfer the stuffing to a large bowl and allow it to cool for 5 minutes. Add the egg white and mix well.

Using a spoon, fill the hollowed zucchini halves with the stuffing, pressing gently to make sure it fills the whole cavity. Set the stuffed zucchinis in the same pan and add the remaining ¾ cup broth. Cover the pan and simmer until the zucchinis are tender, about 20 minutes.

Meanwhile, prepare the avgolemono sauce: Heat a small saucepan over low heat. In a small bowl, beat the egg yolks until frothy, then transfer to the saucepan. Slowly whisk in the lemon juice, followed by a stream of the hot—but not boiling—chicken broth. Whisk constantly over low heat until the sauce thickens, 3 to 5 minutes.

Plate the stuffed zucchini and glaze them with the sauce. Drizzle the zucchinis with the olive oil and sprinkle them with sea salt. Garnish with feta cheese if desired.

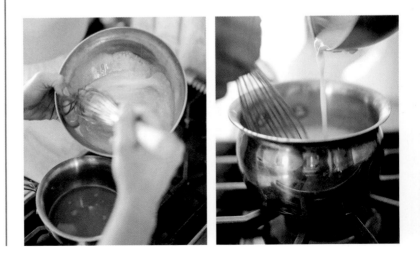

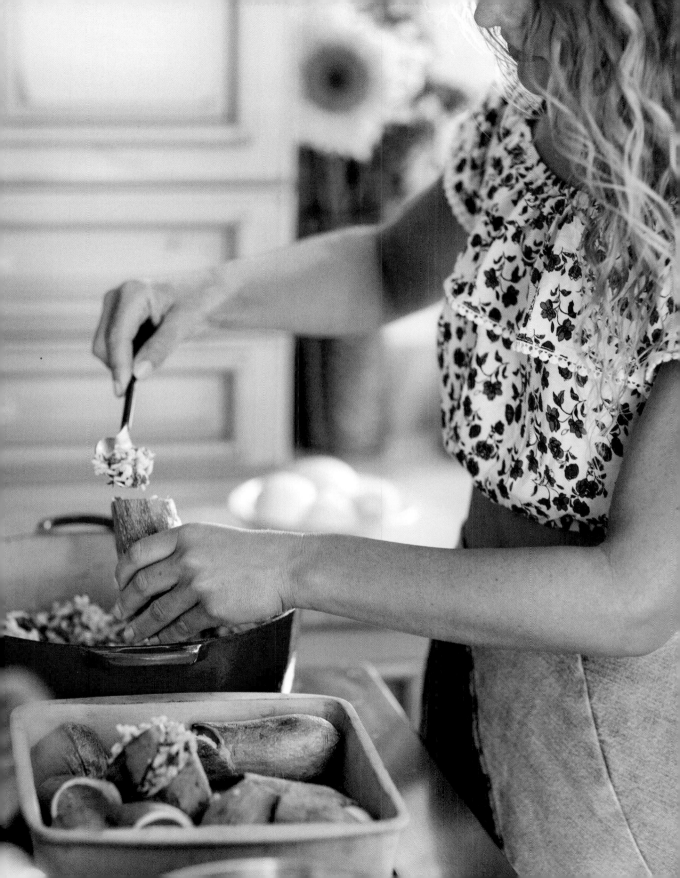

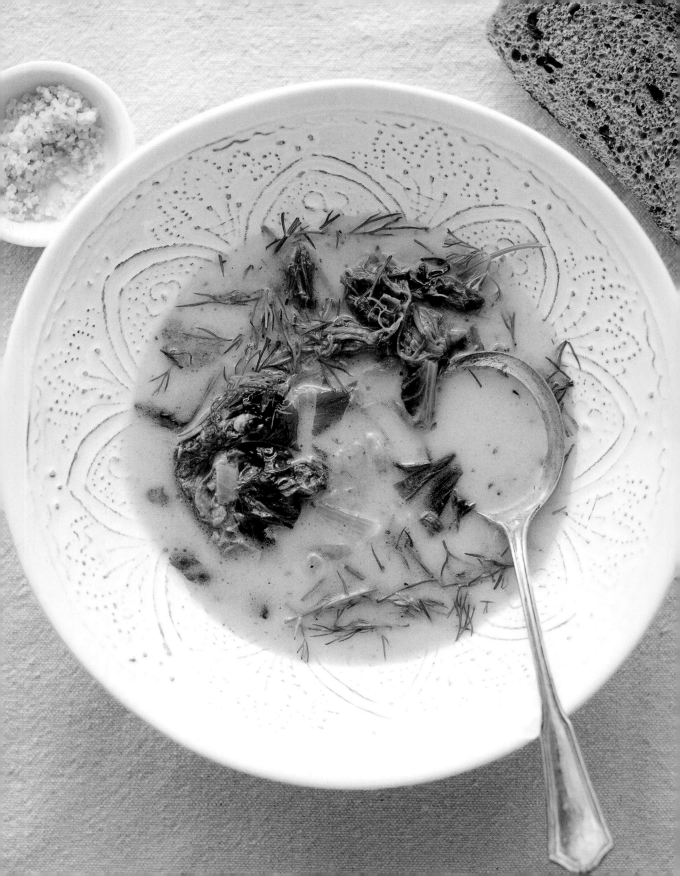

FRICASSEE

Sweet Onion · Dill · Scallions

Serves 4

For the Lamb:

1 tablespoon extra-virgin olive oil

4 lamb shanks, about 1 pound each

1 tablespoon unsalted butter

1 sweet onion, finely chopped

8 cups Mineral-Rich Bone Broth (page 176) or store-bought low-sodium chicken stock

4 heads romaine lettuce, coarsely chopped

4 whole scallions, cut into 1-inch pieces

½ cup chopped fresh dill

Celtic sea salt and freshly ground black pepper

For the Avgolemono Sauce:

4 large egg yolks

Juice of 1 lemon

1 cup Mineral-Rich Bone Broth (page 176) or store-bought low-sodium chicken stock, warmed

Celtic sea salt and freshly ground black pepper

My grandmother Stella's specialty was a fricassee, meat stewed in a rich, egg-based sauce that old wives' tales claim contributes to better health and immunity. In the winter she would make the stew heavier and more fortified with egg yolks, and in the summer she would make it more like a light broth with extra lemon and romaine lettuce.

wild bonus: This recipe includes a gelatin-rich bone broth, which helps keep the mucous membranes in your gut healthy and supple.

To prepare the lamb: In a large pan, heat the olive oil over medium-high heat. Add the shanks and brown on all sides, about 2 minutes per side. Remove from the heat and set aside.

In a medium soup pot, heat the butter over medium heat, add the onion, and cook for 2 to 3 minutes. When soft, add the shanks and the broth. Bring to a boil, then reduce to a simmer, cover, and cook for 1½ hours, adding water if needed.

When the meat begins to fall off the bone, add the romaine, scallions, and dill. Season with salt and pepper, cover, and cook for 20 minutes. Remove from the heat.

Meanwhile, to make the avgolemono sauce: Heat a small saucepan over low heat. In a small bowl, beat the eggs until frothy, then add to the saucepan. Slowly whisk in the lemon juice, followed by a stream of the hot—but not boiling—broth. Whisk constantly until the sauce thickens, 3 to 5 minutes. Season with salt and pepper to taste.

Pour the sauce over the braised meat and vegetables and allow the flavors to meld for 15 minutes before serving—no reheating necessary!

HERB-SCENTED MEATBALLS

Farro · Meat · Basil · Thyme

Serves 3 to 4

1 cup Italian pearled farro

1 tablespoon unsalted butter, plus more for the baking dish

1 medium red onion, diced

¾ cup chopped fresh flat-leaf parsley

1 teaspoon dried thyme

2 teaspoons Celtic sea salt

1 pound ground turkey, beef, or lamb

1 teaspoon freshly ground black pepper

1 large egg

1 cup dry white wine

1 tablespoon extra-virgin olive oil

Chopped fresh basil or parsley, for serving

Farro is an old-world grain, similar to oats, and can be traced back to the Fertile Crescent. It's high in protein and fiber, and has a nice, firm texture with great nutty flavor. The first time I had farro that was braised in a Tuscan clay pot I was attending a nutrigenomics conference in Montecatini Terme—the area in Italy known for its therapeutic waters. There are certain flavors you just never forget, and this was one of them—nutty, savory, and rich.

Just five years ago, I had to source my farro from specialty shops like Dean & DeLuca or Williams-Sonoma. Now, farro is enjoying a newfound popularity, making it easier to find in most grocery stores. There are two methods for cooking farro: long-cooking and quick-cooking. Quick-cooking requires that you soak the grains overnight.

I typically use turkey for this recipe, so I keep a frozen organic variety in my freezer. Grass-fed beef or pastured lamb also would be perfect.

Serve these hearty meatballs alongside the Rigatoni with Butternut Squash and Basil (page 130) or a simple salad.

wild bonus: The addition of farro—a fiber-packed ancient grain—keeps the dish from getting too meat-heavy while still being super satisfying.

If long-cooking the farro: Rinse and drain the farro. Place it in a large pot and add enough water (or stock) to cover. Bring to a boil, reduce the heat to medium-low, and simmer for 30 minutes. Drain and let cool.

If quick-cooking: Put the farro in a large bowl and add enough water to cover. Let the farro soak in the fridge overnight. Drain, transfer the farro to a large pot, add enough water to cover, and bring to a boil. Cook for approximately 10 minutes. Drain and allow to cool.

Preheat the oven to 350°F. Butter a 9 × 13-inch baking dish.

In a large saucepan, heat the 1 tablespoon butter over medium-high heat. Add the onion and cook until softened, 4 to 6 minutes. Stir in the parsley, thyme, and ½ teaspoon of the salt and cook for 2 minutes. Remove from the heat.

Add the ground meat to the pan along with the pepper and remaining 1½ teaspoons salt and mix thoroughly. Stir in the farro. Let the mixture cool slightly, then stir in the egg.

Using your hands, form the meat mixture into 1-inch meatballs and place them side by side (though not touching) in the baking dish. Carefully pour in the wine. Transfer the dish to the oven and bake, rotating the dish front to back halfway through to ensure even cooking, until an instant-read meat thermometer registers at least 165°F for turkey and 160°F for beef or lamb, about 25 minutes.

Transfer the meatballs to a serving platter, drizzle them with olive oil, top with chopped parsley or basil, and serve.

BRAISED CHICKEN THIGHS FROM AVIGNON

Honey · Lavender · Farro

Serves 3 to 4

I cup low-sodium chicken or vegetable broth

½ cup dry white wine

I tablespoon extra-virgin olive oil

I teaspoon dried thyme

I tablespoon dried organic lavender

2 tablespoons honey

I pound boneless, skinless chicken thighs

Celtic sea salt and freshly ground black pepper

2 cups Italian pearled farro

This elegantly aromatic sauce is guaranteed to become one of your go-to recipes for white meats and fish, especially chicken, sole, and halibut. This recipe blends the taste of Provence with some hearty Italian farro. To capture the French countryside even more vividly, buy a lavender plant so you can use the fresh leaves to infuse even more flavor into the dish.

wild bonus: Chicken is a great source of protein and B vitamins, which help with metabolic efficiency.

Preheat the oven to 350°F.

In a large bowl, combine the broth, wine, olive oil, thyme, lavender, and honey.

Rub the chicken thighs with salt and pepper and arrange them in a baking dish just large enough to hold them in a single layer. Pour the broth mixture into the baking dish; it should almost cover the thighs.

Bake for 20 minutes, then flip the thighs over. Add the farro to the baking dish, making sure it's mixed into the sauce well and there's almost enough to cover the farro; add water if necessary. Cover and bake for another 10 minutes if you prefer farro with a denser consistency, 20 minutes for a softer consistency. Check occasionally to ensure the farro doesn't burn.

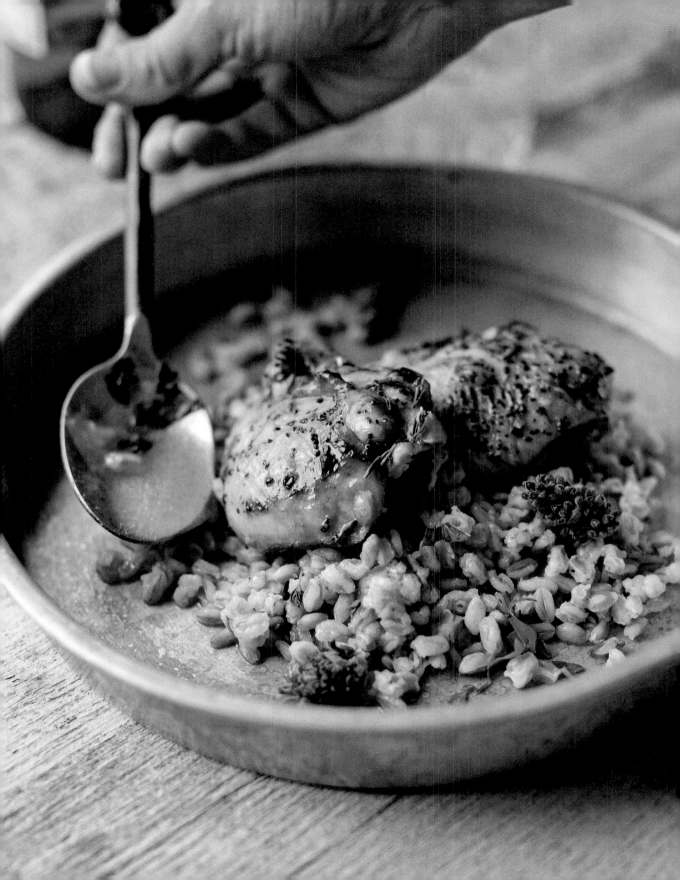

MOUSSAKA

Vegetables · Yogurt · Meat · Garlic · Oregano · Cloves

Serves 6 to 8

2 tablespoons extra-virgin olive oil

2 large eggplants, sliced into ½-inch-thick rounds

6 zucchini, sliced lengthwise

I teaspoon Celtic sea salt

For the Meat Mixture:

I tablespoon extra-virgin olive oil

2 medium onions, thinly sliced

I medium red bell pepper, cut into thin strips

3 garlic cloves, minced

I pound ground lean lamb or beef

I pound chopped plum tomatoes, canned or fresh (seeded, if using fresh)

I½ teaspoons chopped fresh oregano or ½ teaspoon dried

I½ teaspoons chopped fresh thyme or ½ teaspoon dried

I teaspoon ground cinnamon

I teaspoon Celtic sea salt

I can't think of another dish that embodies the healthy yet flavorful recipes of Wild Mediterranean better than moussaka. It features that sweet spot—a 3:I ratio of veggies to protein (maybe even 5:I!)—and cooks together in one dish. The dish can be heavy, though, so I took all the goodness of this classic and made it more biome-friendly.

A few things to note: This dish is traditionally made with lamb, but you can substitute turkey or bison. When purchasing the tomatoes, look for those canned without citric acid and packaged, ideally, in Tetra Pak boxes, or in BPA-free cans.

Preheat the oven to 425°F. Liberally grease 2 large baking sheets with olive oil.

Arrange the eggplant and zucchini slices on the sheets. Drizzle them lightly with olive oil, then sprinkle them with the salt.

Bake the zucchini and eggplant for 10 minutes. Then, using tongs or a spatula, flip them over and bake for another 10 minutes. Remove the vegetables from the oven and place them on paper towels to soak up any excess oil or moisture.

Reduce the oven temperature to 350°F. Lightly oil a 9 × 13-inch baking pan with olive oil.

Meanwhile, prepare the meat mixture: In a large skillet, heat the oil over medium-low heat. Add the onions and cook until they begin to soften, about 2 minutes. Add the bell pepper and sauté until the pepper is soft, another 4 to 5 minutes. Add the garlic and cook for 2 more minutes. Increase the heat to medium-high. Add the ground meat and cook, breaking the meat into fine pieces with your spoon, until cooked through,

½ teaspoon freshly
    ground black pepper

¼ teaspoon freshly
    grated nutmeg

¼ teaspoon red pepper
    flakes (optional)

For the Yogurt Topping:

I tablespoon extra-virgin
    olive oil

¼ cup almond meal or
    all-purpose flour

I½ cups 2% Greek yogurt

3 eggs, beaten

I tablespoon freshly
    grated Pecorino
    Romano or Parmesan
    cheese, plus more for
    serving, if desired

10 to 15 minutes. Drain off any excess fat. Mix in the tomatoes, parsley, oregano, thyme, pepper, cinnamon, salt, black pepper, nutmeg, and red pepper flakes (if using). Simmer for 10 minutes, stirring frequently, then remove the mixture from the heat.

Spread the zucchini slices to cover the bottom of the prepared baking pan. Spread half of the meat mixture over the zucchini. Next, layer on half of the eggplant, making sure to cover the entire pan. Spread the remaining meat mixture over the eggplant. Complete the layering with the remaining eggplant. Set aside.

To make the yogurt topping: In a small bowl, combine the olive oil, almond meal, and yogurt and mix well until combined. Whisk in the eggs and mix until the ingredients form a sauce-like consistency.

Spread the yogurt mixture over the eggplant layer and sprinkle with the cheese.

Bake until golden brown, 50 to 60 minutes. Let the dish rest for 20 minutes before serving. If desired, top the moussaka with additional cheese before serving.

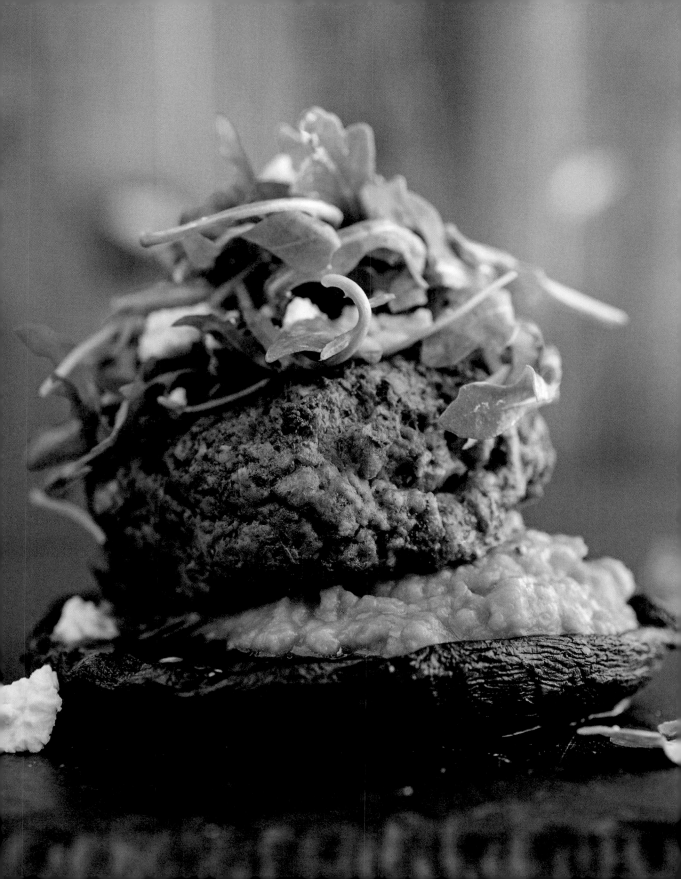

BURGER WITH WHIPPED POTATOES

Sweet Potato · Portobello · Chèvre

Serves 2

I medium sweet potato

2 teaspoons extra-virgin olive oil, plus more as needed

8 ounces ground beef, formed into 2 patties

Celtic sea salt and freshly ground black pepper

2 portobello mushrooms, stems removed

½ cup arugula leaves

¼ cup crumbled chèvre or feta cheese

It's always worth repeating that the main nutritional idea behind the Wild Mediterranean diet is to work an abundance of vegetables into your meals, ideally in a 3:I ratio to meat. This recipe is a perfect example of that balance with the combination of root vegetables and portobello mushrooms (in place of a traditional white-flour bun), plus the meat. If you have access to pastured beef, that's great. If not, you can find quality hormone-free burger patties in the frozen section of the supermarket.

wild bonus: Mushrooms help support healthy immune and inflammatory responses in the gut.

In a small pot, combine the sweet potato with enough cold water to just cover. Bring to a boil, reduce to a simmer, and cook until the sweet potato is soft and cooked through, about 25 minutes. Drain and set aside.

In a skillet, heat the oil over medium heat. Season the beef patties with salt and pepper and cook until an instant-read thermometer inserted into the center registers at least 160°F, about 6 minutes per side. Transfer to a plate and let them rest.

Add a bit more oil to the pan if needed. Season the mushrooms with salt and pepper, add them to the pan, and cook for about 3 minutes.

Peel the sweet potato and transfer to a medium bowl. Use a fork to mash the potato with a bit of olive oil, salt, and pepper.

To serve, layer each mushroom cap with half of the sweet potato mash, a beef patty, half the arugula, and a sprinkling of chèvre.

BRAISED TURKEY BREAST

Sage · Broth · Onion

Serves 4 to 6

4 carrots, cut into 1-inch pieces

6 celery stalks, cut into 1-inch pieces

1 medium onion, coarsely chopped

⅓ cup extra-virgin olive oil

⅓ cup chopped mixed fresh herbs such as parsley, sage, oregano, rosemary, or thyme

1 bone-in turkey breast (4 to 6 pounds)

½ teaspoon Celtic sea salt

½ teaspoon freshly ground black pepper

2 cups Mineral-Rich Bone Broth (page 176), Roasted Vegetable Stock (page 174), or store-bought low-sodium broth

Simple roasted turkey makes a great foundation for many meals. Keeping the 3:1 ratio in mind, just add three servings of veggies and you have lunch or dinner (or breakfast, if you're really hungry). And making a homemade version is nutritionally far superior to what you'll find at the grocery store (less salt, no additives). But roasting a whole bird isn't always convenient, which is why I love just making the breast. Because turkey breast can be dry, I braise it with herb-infused stock, giving it a turn about halfway through cooking to make sure all those juices permeate the skin, and then one last turn to help the meat get golden brown. Layering the cooking liquid with carrots, celery, and onions plus a mix of fresh herbs—any combination of parsley, sage, oregano, and rosemary—adds extra flavor to the meat. Strain and save the cooking liquid to make gravy or to boost the flavor of your next stock.

wild bonus: Most processed deli meats contain nitrates and fillers, so I recommend instead using thin slices of this turkey for sandwiches, layering it on your favorite sprouted bread for a healthier, more gut-friendly alternative.

Preheat the oven to 375°F.

In a medium soup pot, clay pot, or Dutch oven, combine the carrots, celery, and onion. Set aside.

In a small bowl, mix the olive oil with the herbs and toss to coat. Gently lift the skin of the turkey breast and, using your fingers, slide about one-third of the herb/oil mixture underneath. Use the rest to coat the entire breast. Season with the salt and pepper.

Place the turkey breast on top of the vegetables in the pot skin-side up. Pour the broth around the turkey, but not over it. Cover the pot and transfer it to the oven. Bake for 45 minutes. Use tongs to turn the turkey over and bake for another 30 minutes. Turn the turkey once more, uncover, and continue baking until the meat is golden brown and an instant-read thermometer inserted into the thickest part of the breast registers 165°F, another 20 minutes.

Let the turkey rest for about 10 minutes before serving. Strain the cooking liquid, discarding the vegetables, and save to make gravy, stock, or soup.

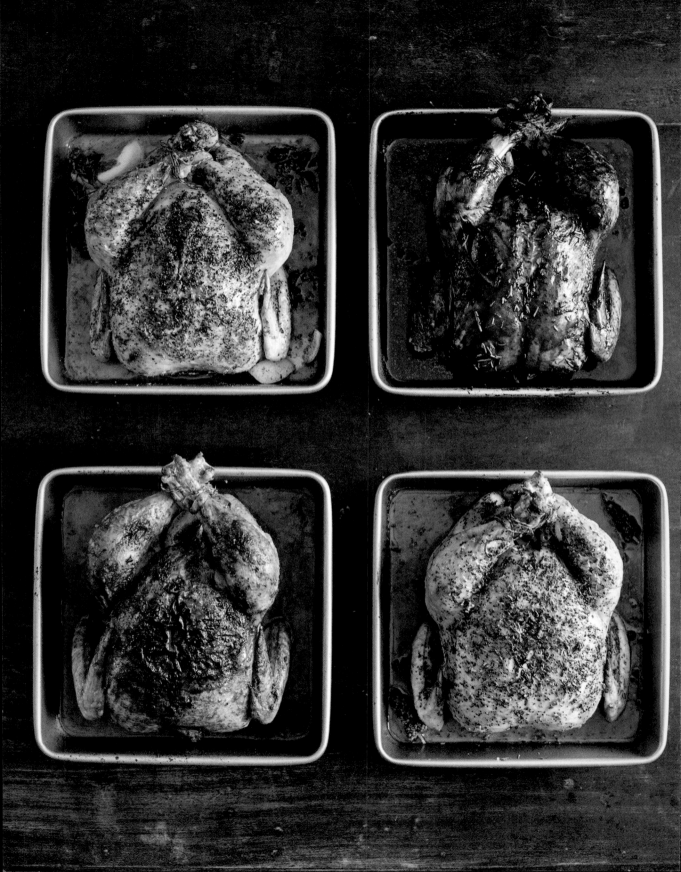

FOUR COUNTRIES, FOUR WAYS: ROAST CHICKEN

Roasted chicken is a versatile foundation for many different meals and every home cook should have a good roast chicken in her repertoire—one that's golden brown, tender, and most important, moist all the way through. The challenge for roasting a whole bird is making sure the leaner white meat stays juicy while the dark meat cooks through. From experience, I've discovered these secrets to getting the most delicious chicken, every time: Stuff your bird with lemons to infuse flavor from the inside out; truss the legs (or tie them together) to help the bird keep its shape and cook evenly; start roasting at 450°F for the first 15 minutes before turning the oven down to 350°F, which will help crisp the skin; and lastly, don't hold back on flavor! The four herb and spice variations that follow are anything but basic!

BASIC ROAST CHICKEN

1 whole (3-pound) chicken

2 lemons, cut into quarters

2 cups water

Chopped root vegetables, such as potatoes or carrots (optional)

Flavor rub (see the variations, page 158) or Celtic sea salt and freshly ground black pepper

Preheat the oven to 450°F.

Remove the giblets from inside the chicken cavity. Discard or reserve for stock.

Insert the lemon quarters into the chicken's front and back cavities. Using kitchen twine, tie the legs together at the "ankle." Trim any excess string to prevent it from burning. To keep the tips of the wings from burning, either tuck them beneath the bird or wrap them in foil.

Add the water to the bottom of a roasting pan. If desired, add chopped vegetables.

Season the entire bird with the flavor rub of your choice or season simply with salt and pepper. Place the bird in the roasting pan breast-side up.

Roast for 30 minutes, then use a large spoon, pastry brush, or baster to baste the chicken with the pan juices. Continue basting every 20 minutes until the chicken is golden brown and cooked through, or an instant-read thermometer inserted in the thigh (and not touching the bone) registers 170°F, about 1 hour (if using a bigger bird, allow another 10 minutes for each additional ½ pound). Any juices that run out should be clear. If still pink, return the chicken to the oven for another 10 minutes and recheck.

Let the chicken rest for at least 15 minutes before slicing and serving.

(recipe continues)

ITALIAN-INSPIRED RUB

Balsamic · Espresso · Rosemary

For a 3-pound chicken:

½ cup balsamic vinegar

I tablespoon extra-virgin olive oil

I tablespoon butter, melted

2 tablespoons instant coffee powder

I tablespoon dark brown sugar

I teaspoon dried rosemary

Celtic sea salt and freshly ground black pepper,
    to taste

In a small bowl, combine all the ingredients
and apply to the chicken before roasting.

GREEK-STYLE RUB

Lemon · Oregano · Garlic

For a 3-pound chicken:

I tablespoon extra-virgin olive oil

I tablespoon butter, melted

I teaspoon garlic powder

2 tablespoons dried Greek oregano

Celtic sea salt and freshly ground black pepper,
    to taste

6 lemon slices

In a small bowl, combine the olive oil, butter,
garlic powder, oregano, and a pinch of salt
and pepper and apply to the chicken. Lay
the chicken in the roasting pan and layer the
lemon slices over the bird.

PROVENÇAL-STYLE RUB

Lemon Zest · Thyme · Pepper

For a 3-pound chicken:

I tablespoon extra-virgin olive oil

I tablespoon butter, melted

2 tablespoons herbes de Provence

2 teaspoons grated lemon zest

Celtic sea salt and freshly ground black pepper,
    to taste

In a small bowl, combine all the ingredients
and apply to the chicken before roasting.

SPANISH-STYLE RUB

Paprika · Garlic

For a 3-pound chicken:

I tablespoon extra-virgin olive oil

I tablespoon butter, melted

2 tablespoons smoked paprika

I teaspoon garlic powder

In a small bowl, combine all the ingredients
and apply to the chicken before roasting.

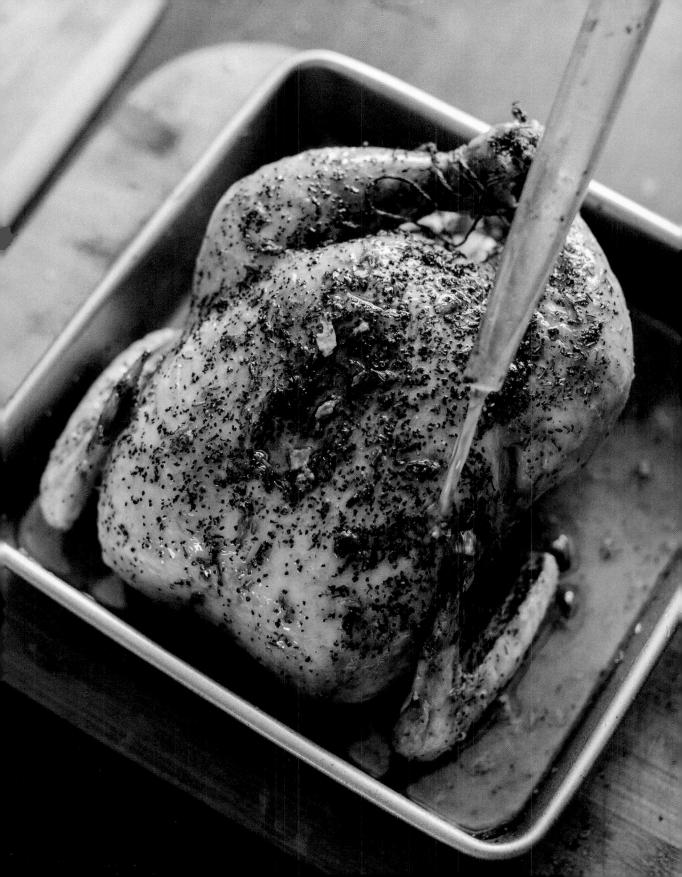

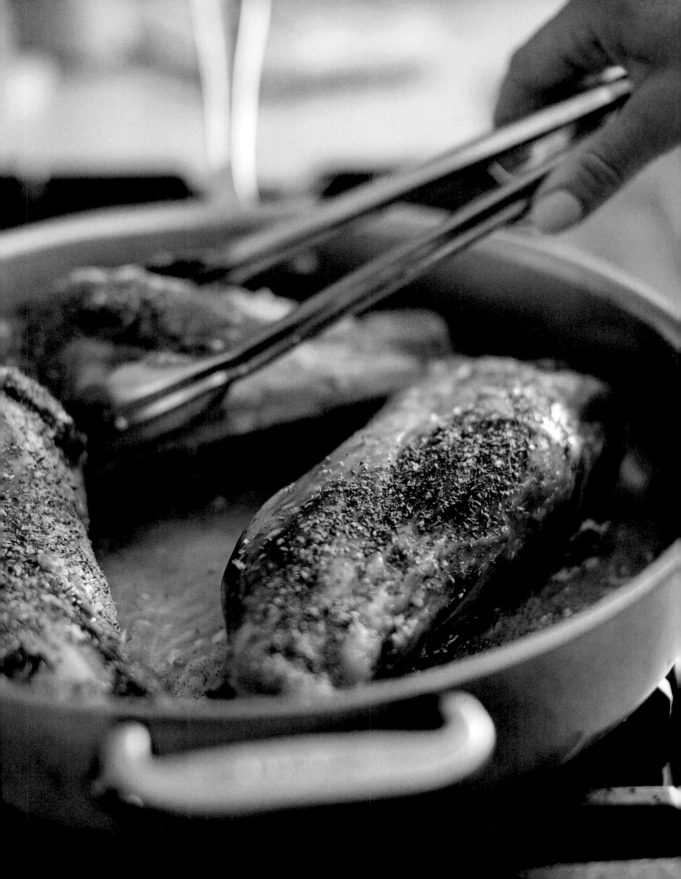

FOUR COUNTRIES, FOUR WAYS: **BRAISED MEAT**

Braising is a simple cooking method that creates a ton of flavor with very little effort. It also coaxes a tender texture from the toughest cuts of meat. At its most basic, all it requires is browning meat and some aromatic vegetables, adding liquid (such as water, broth, or wine), and letting it cook low and slow. These recipes can be made using stewing beef, and braise-friendly cuts, such as lamb shanks or bison.

THE BASICS

Preheat the oven to 350°F degrees.

Sear: In a 6-quart Dutch oven, heat the butter over medium-high heat. Pat the meat dry with paper towels and season with salt and pepper. Arrange the meat in the bottom of the pan in a single layer without crowding and sear on each side for 1 to 2 minutes. The meat should be a caramelized brown color all over. Remove the meat from the pan and set aside.

Sauté: Add the sauté ingredients to the pan, reduce the heat to medium, and cook until the vegetables are softened, 2 to 3 minutes.

Deglaze: Add the deglazing ingredients to the pan and use your spoon to scrape up all the caramelized bits from the bottom of the pan. Bring the liquid in the pan to a boil, then reduce to a simmer.

Braise: Return the meat to the pan along with any additional braising ingredients. Cover and transfer the pan to the oven and cook until the meat is fork-tender, at least 90 minutes, turning the meat halfway through.

(recipe continues)

ITALIAN-STYLE

Chianti · Rosemary · Cocoa · Pearl Onions

Serves 6 to 8

For the Sear:

1 tablespoon butter

3 pounds boneless beef shoulder roast, chuck roast, or top blade, trimmed of excess fat and cut into 1½- to 2-inch pieces

Celtic sea salt and freshly ground black pepper

For the Sauté:

1 yellow onion, coarsely chopped (about 1 cup)

2 celery stalks, coarsely chopped (about ½ cup)

2 carrots, coarsely chopped (about ⅔ cup)

5 garlic cloves, minced

For the Deglaze:

3 cups water

1 cup dry red wine, such as Chianti

1 tablespoon tomato paste

For the Braise:

3 cups peeled pearl onions

2 ounces dried porcini mushrooms, soaked in 2½ cups warm water until soft, then chopped, soaking liquid reserved, strained, and added to the pot

1 tablespoon minced fresh rosemary

1 bay leaf

1 tablespoon unsweetened cocoa powder

GREEK-STYLE

Cognac · Cinnamon · Spring Onions

Serves 6

For the Sear:

1 tablespoon butter

6 small lamb shanks

Celtic sea salt and freshly ground black pepper

For the Sauté:

2 yellow onions, chopped (about 2 cups)

1 carrot, chopped (about ⅓ cup)

For the Deglaze:

3 cups water

¾ cup red wine

⅓ cup Cognac

2 tablespoons red wine vinegar

For the Braise:

1 large tomato, coarsely chopped

1 tablespoon tomato paste

1 bay leaf

1 teaspoon ground cinnamon

Pinch of freshly grated nutmeg

SPANISH-STYLE

Peppers · Olives · Tempranillo

Serves 6 to 8

For the Sear:

1 tablespoon butter

3 pounds boneless beef shoulder roast, chuck roast, or top blade, trimmed of excess fat and cut into 1½- to 2-inch pieces

Celtic sea salt and freshly ground black pepper

For the Sauté:

2 medium onions, halved and thinly sliced (about 2 cups)

3 garlic cloves, chopped

3 medium carrots, diced (about ¾ cup)

2 large red bell peppers, cut in 1¼-inch-wide strips

For the Deglaze:

3 cups water

1 cup dry red wine, such as a Tempranillo

For the Braise:

¼ cup black olives, pitted and chopped

¼ cup green olives, pitted and chopped

1 pound red tomatoes, chopped

2 bay leaves

FRENCH-STYLE

Baby Carrots · Orange Zest · Beaujolais

Serves 6 to 8

For the Sear:

1 tablespoon butter

3 pounds boneless beef shoulder roast, chuck roast, or top blade, trimmed of excess fat and cut into 1½- to 2-inch pieces

Celtic sea salt and freshly ground black pepper

For the Sauté:

3 shallots, thinly sliced

2 celery stalks, thinly sliced (about ½ cup)

2 carrots, thinly sliced (about ⅔ cup)

3 garlic cloves, chopped

For the Deglaze:

2 cups water

3 cups dry red wine, such as Beaujolais

For the Braise:

16 ounces baby carrots (about 3 cups)

2 tablespoons finely chopped fresh flat-leaf parsley leaves

Grated zest of 1 large unwaxed orange (about 2 teaspoons)

MAINS FROM THE SEA

——

The medieval philosopher Maimonides said "Give a man a fish and you feed him for a day; teach a man to fish and you feed him for a lifetime." That's why the ocean symbolizes so much of what's great about the Mediterranean diet and lifestyle. For centuries, the bountiful seas of the region have provided villagers with delicious and healthy foods that are a mainstay of their meals; fortunately, some of the most delicious dishes we can make are also the best for us!

LEMONY FISH
WRAPPED IN GRAPE LEAVES

Lemon · Oregano · Olive Oil

Serves 3 to 4

I pound halibut, snapper, or sea bass

5 tablespoons extra-virgin olive oil

20 brine-packed grape leaves, drained and soaked in water for I hour

Grated zest and juice of I lemon

Celtic sea salt and freshly ground black pepper

Lemon wedges, for serving

This is a good example of taking some of the sea-tox ingredients from Chapter 3 and turning them into a proper main dish. If you can't locate quality halibut, other good options include sole, mahi mahi, and snapper—all low-mercury fish. (Remember that mercury is highly toxic, especially to the nervous system.) While my grandparents could pluck fresh grape leaves off a tree, here in the US, I use the kind that comes in a jar.

wild bonus: Grape leaves are a great source of plant fiber and when paired with omega-3–rich fish and EVOO, are a potent inflammation reliever.

Portion the fish into 4 equal pieces. Lay the fillets on a plate, cover with plastic, and refrigerate while you prepare the grape leaves.

Coat the bottom of a 9 × 13-inch baking dish with a thin layer of olive oil (about 1 tablespoon). Set aside.

Drain the grape leaves. Snip off any protruding stems and discard, then pat the leaves dry with a paper towel. Stack 5 leaves on a cutting board and place a piece of fish in the middle. Season with the lemon zest, a sprinkle of lemon juice, sea salt, pepper, and 1 tablespoon olive oil.

Wrap the leaves completely around the fillet, tucking the edges under the fish as you set it in the baking dish. Repeat with the remaining grape leaves and fillets. Bake until the fish is cooked through and opaque, about 20 minutes. Serve with lemon wedges.

FOUR COUNTRIES, FOUR WAYS: FISH IN PARCHMENT

Serves 2

Fish is a major staple of the Mediterranean diet and cooking en papillote (French for "in a parcel") is one the best ways to prepare it. It's an easy way to make a quick weeknight dinner that's also elegant enough for guests, who should be presented with their own set of scissors to cut open the cute little packages. The fragrant aroma that escapes when the package is opened is reason enough to try it. This method works well for salmon and mild-flavored white fish such as snapper and cod.

To ensure thorough cooking, select fish fillets that are less than I inch thick. And while this technique works best with parchment paper, you can also use foil, though it may react with the vinegar or wine, but don't use wax paper as it will get too gummy.

Try all five flavor variations or come up with some of your own once you've mastered the technique.

You'll need two 12 x 12-inch pieces of parchment. Try to find the unbleached variety on the roll, if possible.

wild bonus: Eating a diet rich in fish—especially fish from clean, sustainable sources—is nourishing not only for your gut, but also for your neurological system.

THE BASICS

Preheat the oven to 425°F.

Fold two 12-inch square sheets of parchment paper in half. Unfold the sheets and brush one side with the olive oil. Arrange the fish and vegetable(s) on the oiled part of each sheet. Top with herbs and/or seasonings. Dot everything with small dabs of butter. Fold the top of the parchment over the fish and crimp the edges together all the way around, making sure it's tightly closed. Place the parcels on a baking sheet and bake for 15 minutes. Remove the parcels from the oven and allow them to rest for a few moments before opening.

ITALIAN-STYLE SALMON

Cherry Tomatoes · Parsley · Orange Zest

I teaspoon extra-virgin olive oil

2 salmon fillets skinless (6 ounces each)

6 to 8 cherry tomatoes, halved

I tablespoon chopped fresh parsley

I teaspoon grated orange zest

A few grinds of black pepper

I teaspoon unsalted butter

PROVENÇAL-STYLE SOLE

Shallot · Fennel · Butter

I teaspoon extra-virgin olive oil

2 sole fillets (3 to 4 ounces each)

I shallot, thinly sliced

I tablespoon finely chopped fresh fennel

2 fresh marjoram or thyme sprigs

¼ teaspoon Celtic sea salt

A few grinds of black pepper

I teaspoon unsalted butter

BASQUE-STYLE COD

Red Bell Peppers · Chickpeas · Sweet Paprika

I teaspoon extra-virgin olive oil

2 cod, snapper, or other mild white fish fillets
    (5 or 6 ounces each)

¼ cup chopped red bell peppers

⅓ cup cooked chickpeas or drained and rinsed
    canned

I teaspoon sweet paprika

I teaspoon Celtic sea salt

A few grinds of black pepper

I teaspoon unsalted butter

Lemon wedges, for serving

GREEK-STYLE SEA BASS

Baby Potatoes · Lemon Zest · Oregano

I teaspoon extra-virgin olive oil

2 sea bass fillets (5 or 6 ounces each)

3 or 4 extra-small baby potatoes

I teaspoon dried oregano

Grated zest from I unwaxed lemon

I teaspoon unsalted butter

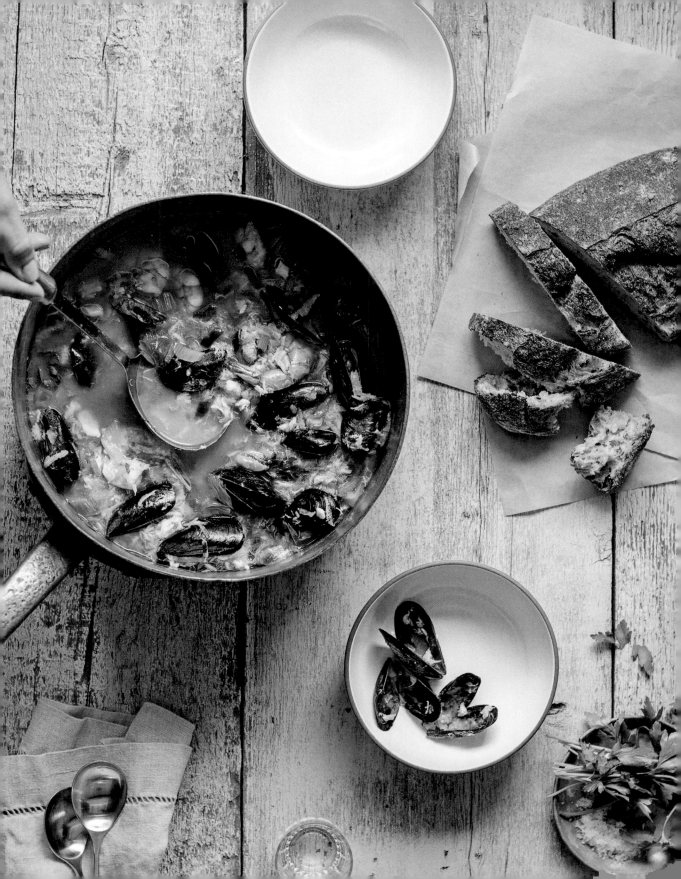

EVERYONE'S FISH STEW

Fennel · Celery · White Wine · Thyme

Serves 4 to 6

- 1 teaspoon unsalted butter
- 1 red onion, thinly sliced
- 3 celery stalks, thinly sliced
- 2 garlic cloves, chopped
- 1 small fennel bulb, trimmed, cored, and thinly sliced
- 8 cups fish stock, homemade (page 175) or store-bought
- 2 cups dry white wine
- 1 medium butternut squash, peeled, seeded, and coarsely grated
- 1 pound salmon fillet, skinless, cut into bite-size pieces
- 1 pound halibut or sole fillet, skinless, cut into bite-size pieces
- 1 pound mussels or littleneck clams, well scrubbed
- 1 pound shrimp, peeled and deveined
- ½ pound sea scallops or langoustines, peeled
- ½ cup chopped fresh flat-leaf parsley
- Grated zest of 1 unwaxed orange
- 1 teaspoon fresh thyme
- Celtic sea salt and freshly ground black pepper
- Extra-virgin olive oil

All Mediterranean countries have their own traditional versions of fish stew. There's French bouillabaisse, Italian cioppino, and Catalan *zarzuela de mariscos*. While these staples of seaside villages all share similar traits—light, bright broths that showcase the freshest local seafood—Greek-style *psarosoupa* has a special place in my heart. It connects me to my family, who believed that this soup could boost a child's weakened immune system during the winter months, and chase away the blues. This recipe is one of my secret weapons: It's a powerful detoxifier that also helps teach your taste buds to crave foods that aren't loaded with artificial flavoring. If you don't live somewhere where you can get fresh langoustines, it's okay to use frozen.

wild bonus: Mineral-rich fish broth has been used as a digestive tonic for centuries by cultures around the world.

In a large soup pot, melt the butter over medium-high heat. Add the onion, celery, garlic, and fennel and cook, stirring occasionally, until softened, about 10 minutes. Stir in the fish stock, wine, and butternut squash. Bring to a boil, cover, reduce the heat to medium-low, and simmer for 30 minutes.

Add the salmon and halibut to the pot and cook for 3 minutes. Add the mussels or clams and cook until they've just opened, about 5 minutes. Discard any that have not opened. Add the shrimp and scallops, cooking them until opaque and cooked through, no more than 10 minutes.

Stir in the parsley, orange zest, and thyme. Season the stew with salt, pepper, extra-virgin olive oil to taste.

SWEET SCALLOP SKEWERS

Radicchio · Honey · Salt

Serves 4

12 medium sea scallops (about 1 pound), tough muscle removed

1 medium red onion, cut into chunks

1 head radicchio, leaves separated

1 tablespoon unsalted butter, plus more if needed

2 tablespoons organic honey

3 tablespoons extra-virgin olive oil

Celtic sea salt and freshly cracked black pepper

If you could wrap up all the flavors of the Mediterranean into one dish it would be this one. Blending bitter and sweet with the fresh, briny flavor of the sea, this recipe brings me back to the Greek Islands. It's almost effortless to make. The great thing about scallops is that they're low in mercury and rich in the quality proteins I recommend in the sea-tox. Remove the tough little side muscle from each scallop before skewering.

wild bonus: Radicchio, a bitter green, is part of the chicory family. This family of greens has been studied for its ability to replenish and balance gut bacteria.

Thread the scallops, onion chunks, and radicchio leaves alternately onto four 12-inch skewers.

In a large cast-iron pan or grill pan, heat the butter over medium-high until very hot but not smoking. Working in batches if necessary, add the skewers and cook, flipping once, until the scallops are golden brown and just cooked through, about 2 minutes per side. If needed, add a tiny bit more butter between batches so the scallops do not stick to the pan. Transfer the skewers to a large plate.

In a small saucepan, gently warm the honey and olive oil over low heat. Season with salt and cracked pepper. Drizzle the sauce over the skewers and serve immediately.

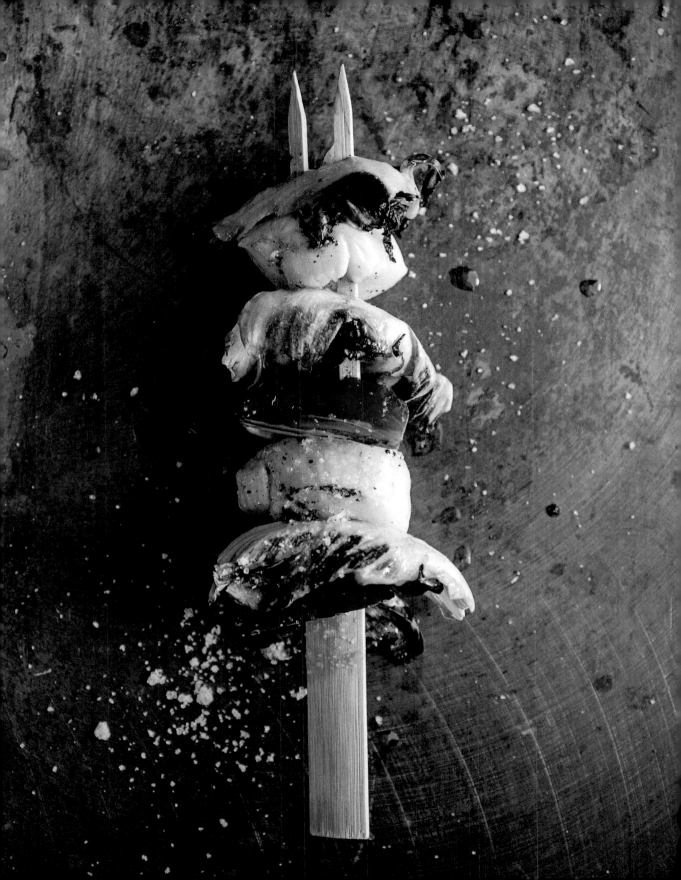

STAPLES & BASICS

The best kitchens aren't those with fancy appliances or the newest color schemes. Their secret is a well-stocked pantry. The stocks and vinaigrette in this short but essential section will become mainstays of your new approach to cooking, bringing better quality and superior flavor to even simple salads, soups, and braises. In every way they are worth the expense and time required to make them.

WILD VINAIGRETTE

You'll soon consider this your go-to vinaigrette. It's simple and flavorful, and incredibly versatile. Using a basic ratio, you can easily mix and match ingredients to create flavors that suit whatever you're eating. What makes it particularly suited to experimentation is the addition of cold-pressed juice. Now that most grocery stores carry a wide selection of bottled options, you can concoct any number of variations. Want a fancy "gourmet" vinaigrette like raspberry or blueberry? Whisk together fruit juice with a little champagne vinegar and olive oil. Want an Asian-style vinaigrette? Use ginger, garlic, miso, sesame oil, peanut oil, or soy sauce. An Italian Vinaigrette? Basil, garlic, or simply get creative! See the Resources section (page 209) for a list of my favorite brands of oils and vinegars.

wild bonus: Including healthy fats with vegetables helps to increase their nutritional value.

Basic Ratio:

1 part acid
+
2 parts
cold pressed juice
+
3 parts oil

vinaigrette

ACIDS: Vinegar (coconut, apple cider, balsamic, or rice) or citrus juice (lemon, lime, or grapefruit)

COLD-PRESSED JUICES: Look for those with a medley of fruits and vegetables, roots, citrus, and greens

OILS: Extra-virgin olive oil, nut/seed oils (hazelnut, walnut, flaxseed, pistachio, or sunflower), coconut oil, avocado oil

Salt and freshly ground black pepper

In a medium bowl, combine the acid and juice. Slowly drizzle in the oil while constantly whisking. Season with salt and pepper to taste. Congratulations, you just made a vinaigrette!

Extra Credit

If you want a slightly thicker vinaigrette—and one that won't separate in the fridge—add an emulsifier such as an egg yolk or a small dollop of mayonnaise or mustard before you drizzle in the oil. Just be mindful that consuming a raw egg may increase your risk of foodborne illness.

Always taste the vinaigrette with a leaf or two of the greens it will be dressing, so you know what it will actually taste like on the plate. Some lettuces can suck up the acid tang, others amplify. Adjust the ingredients to your satisfaction and serve.

ROASTED VEGETABLE STOCK

Makes about 8 cups

You would be well advised to keep a few quarts of this stock in your freezer. Roasting the vegetables before making the stock gives it earthy, smoky flavor that lends depth to just about anything, from soups to braising liquids to cooking beans and grains.

wild bonus: This broth is a digestive tonic that helps infuse the gut with minerals.

8 carrots, coarsely chopped

10 mushrooms, such as white button or cremini, trimmed

3 onions, coarsely chopped

2 leeks, white and light green parts only, halved, well washed, and coarsely chopped

2 garlic cloves, peeled but whole

Extra-virgin olive oil

Sea salt and freshly ground black pepper

12 cups water

1 cup dry white wine

2 fresh thyme sprigs

Handful of fresh parsley sprigs

2 bay leaves

4 black peppercorns

Preheat the oven to 375°F

Arrange the carrots, mushrooms, onions, leeks, and garlic on a large rimmed baking sheet in a single layer. Drizzle the vegetables with olive oil and season with salt and pepper.

Roast the vegetables until tender and beginning to caramelize, about 40 minutes, turning after 20 minutes. Scrape the vegetables into a stockpot.

Add the water, wine, thyme, parsley, bay leaves, and peppercorns to the vegetables. Cover and bring the mixture to a boil over medium-high heat. Reduce to a simmer and cook for 1½ hours. Strain the stock through a cheesecloth-lined sieve into a bowl and cool (discard the solids). Transfer to 1-quart containers and store in the fridge for up to 2 days or the freezer for up to 6 months.

FISH STOCK

Makes 8 to 10 cups

1 large leek

2 pounds fish heads or bones from nonoily white fish such as sea bass, gills removed

1 tablespoon unsalted butter

1 medium white onion, chopped

2 carrots, chopped

2 celery stalks, chopped

½ bulb fennel, chopped

2 bay leaves

Handful fresh flat-leaf parsley sprigs

15 fresh thyme sprigs

1 teaspoon ground cinnamon

1 teaspoon fennel seeds

2 cups dry white wine

Adding fish stock is the best way to deepen the flavors of any seafood dish you're cooking. It's just as easy as vegetable stock to make and less than 45 minutes of cooking time, compared to the hours bone broth needs. Although you can, of course, buy ready-made fish stock at the store, I recommend seeking out fishmongers or grocers who butcher their own whole fish. They're usually more than happy to sell you their scraps. I'm fortunate to have a friendly neighborhood restaurant nearby that always has fish heads to spare, especially from sea bass, which are particularly flavorful.

wild bonus: Including this broth in your cooking rotation helps infuse the gut with the mineral-rich properties of the sea.

Trim the leek of its dark green leaves and roots and cut it into quarters lengthwise. Submerge the pieces in a large bowl of water and agitate to remove any grit. Allow them to sit while you prepare the fish and sautéed vegetables.

Rinse the fish heads, making sure there is no trace of gills or blood. Set aside.

In a large (12-quart) stockpot, melt the butter over medium heat. Add the onion, carrots, celery, and fresh fennel and sauté until soft, 4 to 5 minutes. Add the fish heads, bay leaves, parsley, thyme, cinnamon, fennel seeds, and wine. Lift the leek pieces out of the water and add to the pot. Pour in enough water to cover the solids by at least 3 inches, but no so much that it will boil over. Reduce the heat to low, cover, and simmer for 30 minutes.

Allow the stock to cool before straining through a cheesecloth-lined sieve into a bowl (discard the solids). Transfer to 1-quart containers and store in the fridge for up to 2 days or in the freezer for up to 6 months.

MINERAL-RICH BONE BROTH

Makes about 8 cups

I to 2 pounds lamb, beef, or chicken bones

2 large onions, chopped

4 garlic cloves, minced

5 celery stalks, chopped

3 carrots, chopped

3 fresh thyme sprigs

I fresh rosemary sprig

2 bay leaves

½ cup chopped fresh flat-leaf parsley

I tablespoon apple cider vinegar

Pinch of sea salt

Note: I usually schedule a broth-making day every month or so and stock the freezer so I always have some on hand. Make sure to label the type of broth clearly if you're making different varieties—I once accidentally used a fish broth for a hearty beef stew!

Nutrient-rich bone broth is a restorative, curative, and essential ingredient in almost every cuisine around the world, and it's no different in Mediterranean cooking. While the recipes differ from country to country, they all result in deeply flavored, nutrient-dense broth that's just as delicious to sip as it is to use in your everyday cooking. I recommend lamb as the base, but beef and pastured chicken are also delicious. Always buy whole organic chickens, so you can save the bones after you've roasted and eaten the meat. Just store the bones in the freezer until you have enough to make stock. Roasting the bones before simmering them gives this broth even deeper flavor.

wild bonus: This gelatin-rich broth helps protect the gut and its mucous membrane.

Preheat the oven to 400°F.

Scatter the bones in a roasting pan. Roast until the bones are browned, 45 minutes to 1 hour. Transfer the bones to a large pot.

Add the remaining ingredients and add water to cover (about 10 cups). Bring to just under a boil and reduce the heat. Simmer for 2 hours, skimming occasionally to remove any fat or foam that rises to the surface.

Strain the broth through a fine-mesh sieve (discard the solids).

Let the broth cool to room temperature and transfer to 1-quart containers. Store in the refrigerator for up to 2 days or freezer for up to 6 months.

MOM'S SECRET TZATZIKI

Serves 8

3 medium cucumbers, seeded

2 cups full-fat Greek yogurt

2 cups kefir

I cup extra-virgin olive oil

2 tablespoons finely chopped fennel

2 tablespoons chopped fresh dill

2 tablespoons chopped fresh mint

I tablespoon chopped fresh flat-leaf parsley

I tablespoon crushed garlic (about I clove)

I tablespoon fresh lemon juice

I tablespoon ouzo

Sea salt and ground white pepper, to taste

A tzatziki recipe is to a Greek cook like red sauce is to an Italian—every family has its own, and you'll never taste exactly the same one twice.

It might seem like a simple condiment, but it's all about getting the right balance of flavors from fresh herbs like dill, mint, and parsley plus spicy garlic and sweet fennel.

How much garlic or cucumber you use really comes down to personal preference. Just make sure that the cucumber is seeded and drained of all its natural water, or else the consistency will be too loose. As with any recipe in which the ingredients are raw, quality is key.

wild bonus: Garlic and its disease-preventing properties is the real star of this dish.

Peel the cucumbers and grate them on the coarse holes of a box grater. Place the grated cucumber in a sieve and gently press out the liquid. Transfer to a medium bowl.

Add all the remaining ingredients and season to taste. Refrigerate overnight before serving to let the flavors meld.

A LITTLE SOMETHING SWEET

——

Who doesn't crave a little something sweet every once in a while? Most dessert recipes from the ancient past used honey from the cook's own hives or molasses made from grapes. Although it's true that a sugar is still a sugar, using a bit of unrefined products like these give a unique depth of flavor, and satisfy our desire for a sweet indulgence in the healthiest way.

CHOCOLATE YOGURT SUNDAE

Serves 1

I cup 2% Greek yogurt

¼ cup semisweet chocolate chips

I tablespoon chopped pecans

I tablespoon coconut flakes (I prefer sweetened, but unsweetened is fine)

½ cup fresh berries (optional)

Greek yogurt might be all the rage now, but ten years ago it was virtually nonexistent in American grocery stores. I, on the other hand, grew up eating Greek-style sheep's milk yogurt on my summer visits to the islands. It was made in the traditional method of fermenting in a clay container—the way it's still sold at most grocers in Greece. I can see why it's caught on here—its tangy flavor combined with a thick, creamy consistency is so much better than the runny, flavorless stuff you normally get in the dairy aisle.

It's also so versatile flavorwise—going sweet or savory depending on what you put in it. It's the perfect base for tzatziki (page 187), but is just as delicious as the foundation for this take on the chocolate-banana sundaes I loved as a kid. The trick is to get the temperature of the yogurt just right—frozen enough that it's like ice cream but not so frozen that it crystallizes.

wild bonus: Polyphenols—which help prevent degenerative diseases such as cancer and heart disease—are abundant in cocoa beans.

Freeze the Greek yogurt for 1 hour in a glass or ceramic bowl, stirring once at the 30-minute mark. (This breaks up any ice crystals.) If you prefer a firmer consistency, freeze the yogurt for up to 2 hours.

In a medium glass or metal bowl set over a small saucepan of simmering water, melt the chocolate.

Divide the yogurt between two bowls. Drizzle the chocolate over the yogurt and top with chopped nuts, coconut flakes, and berries (if using).

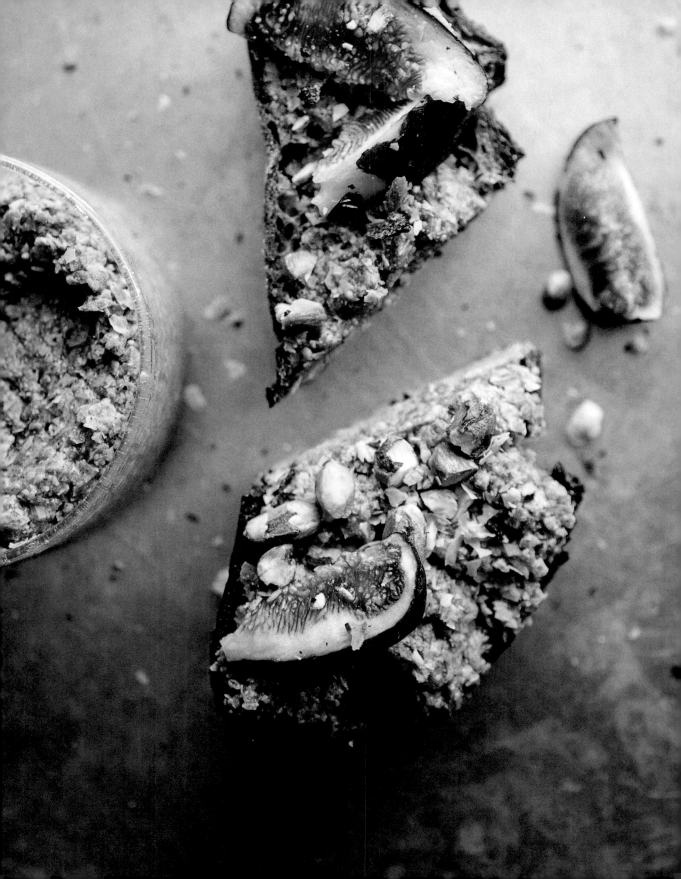

BAKLAVA BUTTER

Makes 1½ cups (about 12 servings)

1¼ cups walnuts

½ cup roasted almonds

⅓ cups pistachios

½ cup almond meal

¼ cup organic honey

1 tablespoon coconut sugar

1 teaspoon ground cinnamon

Pinch of sea salt

1 tablespoon extra-virgin olive oil

1 teaspoon vanilla extract

Yes, you read that right: The nutty, honey-sweetened decadence of Greece's most famous dessert—without all the layers of buttered phyllo dough and heavy syrup. By folding all the ingredients into softened "butter," you get a spreadable guilty pleasure to enjoy on sprouted-grain toast, stirred into yogurt, or stuffed into dates. After all, it's okay to treat yourself once in a while. It's all about balance! This makes quite a bit and should be used within 10 days, so consider sharing some as a gift!

wild bonus: Healthy fats plus nut-derived fiber are essential building blocks for balanced gut health.

In a food processor, combine the walnuts, almonds, and pistachios. Pulse until coarsely ground or finely chopped— be careful not to overprocess. Transfer the mixture to a medium bowl and stir in the almond meal.

In a small pot, combine the honey, sugar, cinnamon, and salt with 2 tablespoons of water. Bring to a gentle simmer over low heat, then remove from the heat and add directly to the bowl with the nut mixture. Add the olive oil and vanilla extract and mix well.

Transfer the butter to a clean glass jar, refrigerate, and use within 1 week.

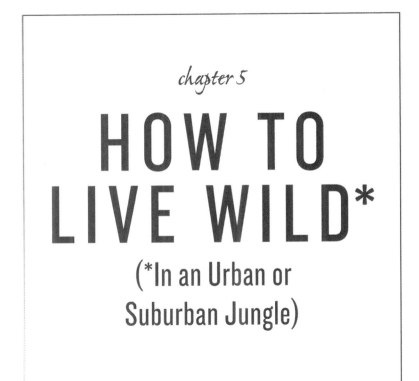

chapter 5

HOW TO LIVE WILD*

(*In an Urban or Suburban Jungle)

"Live in the sunshine.
Swim in the sea.
Drink the wild air."

Ralph Waldo Emerson

FINDING YOUR WILD ISN'T JUST ABOUT WHAT YOU EAT. THOUGH THAT'S A MAJOR PIECE, TAPPING into a lifestyle that brings you joy, satisfaction, and peace is equally important for your well-being. You can't choose one or the other and expect to live a long, healthy life. When I think about my relatives in Greece—from my youngest cousins to my grandparents—what always comes up is how much *fun* they have. And they balance that with finding moments of quiet, connection, and rest. Who needs the gym when you can approach the world with childlike curiosity and a spirit of play? Who needs mood-enhancing drugs when you can get a good night's sleep and have stress-coping outlets? And who needs, well, anything else, when you're part of a community that supports and uplifts you?

Also, bringing the stresses and pleasures of life into balance is necessary for good gut health. Beneficial bacteria surround us all the time. (Especially when we're out in nature, which we'll talk about in much more detail later in this chapter.) Japanese researchers believe that when we breathe in good, clean air, we're also inhaling beneficial bacteria, which in turn produces plant-derived essential oils that fight off harmful microorganisms and negatively charged ions. The more we breathe them in, the happier and healthier we become. These helpful bacteria are referred to collectively as phytoncides, literally "plant-derived extermi-nators," or scrubbing bubbles for our guts. However, these guys can't do their job if your GI tract's circulation turns sluggish. In fact, sitting for long stretches can negatively affect your gut health. To get these microorganisms moving, you have to move, too. Walk, run, jump rope, climb trees, paddle a canoe, dance or whatever you're inclined to do. Moving your body doesn't just burn calories—it keeps your forgotten organ's circulation working properly. Another strong vote for finding a form of exercise you like and doing it often!

Managing stress is also crucial for optimal digestive health. When you let yourself be consumed by worry, anxiety, or overwhelming thoughts, those emotions go directly to your gut. It's true: Your brain and your gut are in conversation with each other. If you need proof of that connection, think about how you feel sensations in your stomach when you experience dread or excitement. Or consider that the very thought of eating can release the stomach's juices before food gets there. This road goes both ways, too. Just as your mood and stress can wreak havoc on your microbiome, an unhealthy microbiome can affect your mood. So it's critically important to find healthy ways to deal with life's demands.

This chapter is devoted to helping you achieve a healthy balance with your gut, from the outside in, whether it's finding an enjoyable movement routine, being out in nature, creating a stronger social network, getting a good night's sleep, or even having more sex (most excellent for the gut!). It's time for you to discover the bigger, wider, more wild world that surrounds you and learn how it can help you feel healthier and more vibrant.

Adopt a Childlike Perspective

A big part of finding your wild—including moving more and adopting a more positive, gut-nurturing outlook—is facing life with an open, imaginative attitude. "The Spaghetti Problem" competition is a great example of how that kind of free-spirited thinking helps us solve problems and feel better about ourselves. It's a seemingly simple exercise designed by Peter Skillman, one of the tech world's leading user-interface designers. Teams are given eighteen minutes to work with two pieces of spaghetti, tape, some string, and a marshmallow. The group that crafts the tallest structure that supports the weight of the marshmallow wins.

Skillman has tested engineers, computer programmers, MBA students, and tech executives. But the most successful group of all? Kindergartners.

The MBAs spent precious time discussing who would take on which roles. The engineers drew up plans and wouldn't let them go even when they didn't work. Invariably, the kindergartners jumped in, tried things, and started failing immediately. Their system was simple: Build, fail. Build again, fail. Rebuild, fail. They didn't plan, they didn't fret about egos. They all just worked together until they succeeded. And they enjoyed themselves while they did it. In the meantime, the "professionals" ended up grumbling and defeated.

Children are fearless. They excel at play and live in a world fueled by imagination and creativity. Kids allow wonder to lead them to endless discoveries. They live in the moment. They aren't afraid to ask foolish questions. They have the capacity for pure joy.

It's hard to retain those qualities in the process of growing into a supposedly sophisticated adult. But the villagers back in my hometown keep that spark of childlike curiosity alive. They argue good-naturedly. They ask questions and express emotions in an authentic, unrestrained way. As a result, they have a healthy aura of youthfulness about them. When they throw parties in their village, everyone dances and sings and no one worries about looking foolish. This ability to be present and in the moment is as much a key to their longevity as eating their daily greens.

> Children are fearless. They excel at play and live in a world fueled by imagination and creativity. Kids allow wonder to lead them to endless discoveries.

I admit, that for a while, I forgot this important lesson myself. Like a lot of people, after I graduated from college, I felt as if I had to fit a certain mold. There's no dearth of love in a big Greek family— whether you live in Greece or in the States—but there are also expectations about how you should behave and what your role should be in life. It took me years to realize that I am still Stella, the little girl who fearlessly gutted a fish at age three, who loved to play in the earth and the sea and asked questions about everything. It was a relief to realize this. In many ways, I feel younger today than I did years ago, in part because I learned to reconnect with that youthful energy and sense of abandon.

You may not see the direct connection between your physical well-being and having a good time, but it's there—because every time you do something that frees your body and your spirit, you're coming that much closer to the health and vitality we all deserve.

FUN AS EXERCISE

I love watching the villagers play beach tennis on the sands of Santorini. It's a whole lineup of guys in everything from teeny Speedos to board shorts, showing off their physiques and strutting their stuff. They range in age from twenty-five to seventy-five years old—and they all look good! Playing hours of tennis, a hugely popular pastime on the beaches of the Mediterranean, keeps them fit. That's a key lesson in finding your wild: Don't look at exercise as a chore. Find a way to play that involves moving your body. If you're bored with your workouts, then change things up! Here are a few ideas to get you started.

BOXING

Boxing provides a great total body workout and requires constant attention. Boxing offers a similar cardio workout to running or cycling. It also taxes your core muscles and is as effective for your midsection as sit-ups or crunches. Plus, it's a great stress-buster after a long day at the office.

FENCING

A sport that could qualify as an art form, fencing involves a lot of footwork and lunges in addition to building up arm muscles. This leads to a workout that develops balance, agility, coordination, strength, and flexibility. Since there's a lot of stopping and starting, fencing is a great interval training sport.

KAYAKING AND STAND-UP PADDLE BOARDING

Kayaking and stand-up paddle boarding (SUP) offer a spectrum of rewards. You get good exercise as you propel yourself along and take in the beauty of nature around you. Both activities are relatively easy to learn, and you can rent the equipment while you try it out. Paddling has the benefit of providing you with some alone time or can be a different kind of fun when you do it with a bunch of friends.

RACQUETBALL

The U.S. Racquetball Association claims that a game of racquetball works every muscle group, and that in a one-hour game, a player can run over two miles. Many health club chains have racquetball courts and will pair you for play with other members. Plus, the equipment needed is minimal: It requires only a racquet, a ball, goggles, and a pair of gloves.

ROCK CLIMBING

Climbing delivers a great cardiovascular workout along with intense upper-body strength-building. It increases your balance and flexibility (since you often find yourself in unusual positions), and requires complete concentration. You can start on a local gym's climbing wall, then graduate to the real thing, where you'll witness some gorgeous natural sights as well.

ROLLERBLADING

Rollerblade faster than ten miles an hour, and you'll get an aerobic workout equal to running. This form of skating builds strength in all of your lower-body muscles, since you use those to push yourself forward and to maintain your balance. Add some challenging uphill paths for a great cardiovascular workout.

SKATEBOARDING

Skateboard regularly to build cardio endurance as well as strengthen your legs and core. Plus it's great for running errands!

SURFING

Surfing provides both aerobic and anaerobic exercise. You have to carry your board in and out of the water, paddle, jump up to balance on the board, swivel your body for turns, and of course, swim. Also, its natural environment, salt water, has healing properties that are great for your skin and reduces inflammation in joints and muscles.

TANGO DANCING

Essentially a walking dance, you can learn to tango at almost any age. It offers a terrific cardiovascular workout as well as improved mobility, balance, stride length, and core strength. Research has shown that dancing can even help to counteract dementia.

TRAMPOLINE

When you jump on a trampoline, you get a cardio workout as well as a great leg, glute, and core exercise. It can also improve your balance and coordination. Plus, you have to love an activity that you can do with your kids!

Just Play

In life, attitude is everything. Kids just want to have fun. Think back to your favorite childhood activities. Mine always involved horses, climbing trees, or swimming with my favorite tunes blaring nearby. Maybe you were in your element singing into a hairbrush or camping in the backyard. Reach back to those moments and access that childhood spirit. Here are some ideas:

- **GO ON ADVENTURES.** Pack a picnic and go for a hike. Take the dog to an off-leash park on the other side of town. Scope out local event listings and hit one you've never been to before, such as an art gallery opening or a planetarium show.

- **DANCE.** Find a local dance night featuring your favorite style of dance—or one you've always wanted to learn. Salsa, anyone? You can always dance at home. One of my very favorite YouTube channels is www.youtube.com/user/DanceTutorialsLIVE, which includes tutorials on dance moves from salsa to traditional Greek dance. *Opa!*

- **SEEK OUT LAUGHTER.** Get friends together for a night at a comedy club. Go on an open-mic night and challenge one another to go on stage.

- **COLOR.** Adult coloring books are all the rage. Feel free to go outside the lines.

- **STARGAZE.** Connect the stars to make images or use the Night Sky app to explore constellations.

- **SING.** Find a place that offers karaoke or add a lip-syncing competition to your next party.

Move More—and Make It Fun

When was the last time you had a good time working out? Or did something simply to find out what your body was capable of? Think about the ways you incorporate exercise in your adult life. Kids get their exercise just by running around the playground, climbing trees, and making endless trips up a ladder for the thrill of riding down a slide. I did that, too. But by the time I got to college, I fell into the "adult" idea of a workout: making monotonous trips to the gym just because I thought I should, hitting plateaus doing the same old routines. I was a personal trainer for a while, so I have nothing against gyms, but after years of working out, don't you sometimes ask yourself, *Why am I doing this?* Now I ask my clients the same thing. Are you doing it just to lose or maintain a certain weight? To be able to check it off a list? What if your exercise involved an activity you *actually looked forward to?* The biggest payoff is that you'll do something you actually like more, which means more circulation-boosting, gut-balancing benefits for you!

Get Out in Nature

Have you noticed that you feel better and healthier when you hike a nature trail or take a seaside stroll? You may have thought it was just being away from an urban center, the calming effect of a beautiful view or the lulling sound of water. But it turns out, scientists believe that getting outside in nature is actually good for your gut, and therefore has a powerful impact on your overall health.

Humans, like animals, gain nutrients from their surroundings by breathing them in or absorbing them through the skin. The GI tract then processes these nutrients. Our surroundings help to feed the "circulation" of our digestive tract by helping to shift nutrients to our organs and cells. Our digestive system takes in nutrients, breaks them down, and delivers them to our organs, then takes away organ waste and disposes of it. This process is so critical that one-fourth of your body's cardiac output is dedicated to your GI tract's circulation.

> Our surroundings help to feed the "circulation" of our digestive tract by helping to shift nutrients to our organs and cells.

Technology can be a wonderful thing, but it can also rob us of elements that contribute to our quality of life in an important way. Humans were not meant to be indoors all day, nor were we intended to sit for long stretches. Yet, the average American spends nearly five hours a day doing just that. So put down your phone. Go outside. Move your body and get your circulation going. Take in a long breath and love your gut.

Manage Your Daily Stress

Stress is tough on every part of your body, including your gut. Yet stress is a constant companion in our industrialized world. The key to stress is not what causes it, but rather how you respond to it. The longest-living people learn to manage their stress in positive ways, which in turn, encourages good digestive health.

In my practice, when clients first come to me, they tell me their responses to stress include binge eating or reaching for junk food, smoking, drinking alcohol to excess, procrastination, sleeping to avoid dealing with issues, or zoning out in front of the TV—all gut busters.

Take my client Robert, who is one of those people who "have everything"—a handsome guy with great wealth, a strong marriage, a healthy family, and a high-powered career that involves a lot of international travel. Like many of my male clients, he is a Type A perfectionist. He leads a highly regimented life, hitting the gym daily and eating the same nutritionally undiverse meals almost every day to closely regulate his caloric intake.

> The longest-living people learn to manage their stress in positive ways, which in turn, encourages good digestive health.

He was referred to me by his doctor, and when I read the results of his GI panel along with his other lab work, I could understand why. The person sitting in front of me looked healthy but internally, something else was going on. His tests showed high levels of C-reactive protein (CRP), which indicated extreme inflammation in the body. When something harmful or irritating affects a part of our body, it triggers a biological response. Inflammation, specifically acute levels, signals that the body is trying to heal itself. In Robert's case, it's possible that his elevated stress levels may have made his immune system less effective because stress itself can elicit an immune response, causing the body to release pro-inflammatory cytokines. And this can lead to dysbiosis, or imbalance in the gut, which has far-reaching negative health implications.

I asked Robert to fill out a survey about his habits. He estimated his stress level as a nine out of ten. When people are that stressed, adjusting diet alone isn't enough.

I told Robert that if he wanted to work with me, he had to make some serious changes to his lifestyle as well.

"When was the last time you did something spontaneous?" I asked.

He looked at me and laughed. Then his face turned serious when he realized he couldn't come up with an answer. I explained my views on the human need for play. As we worked together, he learned he had to modify not only his diet—which we adjusted to include Wild Mediterranean staples, kicked off by a pre-tox and detox—but more important his routine; because if his stress levels continued to soar, then his immune system would continue to suffer, no matter how well he ate. He needed to make having fun a priority. Now he is taking surfing lessons and often goes salsa dancing with his wife. His health is remarkably improved—no medication required.

Stress Busters

Starting the day with something you love to do puts you into a positive frame of mind, which in turn creates a more healthful environment for your digestive system. Play fun music or a compelling audiobook or podcast on your commute rather than listening to the news. The point is to greet the day with the best mind-set possible so you're able to challenge and conquer the world—or at least your small part of it.

Technology is great when it helps you find unique ways to start your day off right. One startup in New York offers an early-morning dance party providing fresh juices, organic espresso, farm-to-table foods and, of course, music. When I first saw the press release, I thought, *This is genius!*

If whatever you choose to do is fun and childlike, then you're on the right track. Here are some possibilities:

CONSIDER GETTING A PET. It's a fact: Dog owners live longer and are happier than non-pet owners. They're less likely to develop heart disease, perhaps because dog owners tend to walk more every day than people who have no pets. Pets calm us and positively impact our metabolic systems. In one study, a group of people with high blood pressure and jobs they described as "very stressful" agreed to adopt a dog or cat. Six months later, they reported feeling significantly less pressure at work. Pets can teach us something special, as John Grogan said so wonderfully in his book *Marley and Me*: "Marley taught me about living each day with unbridled exuberance and joy, about seizing the moment and following your heart. He taught me to appreciate the simple things—a walk in the woods, a fresh snowfall, a nap in a shaft of winter sunlight . . . A dog doesn't care if you're rich or poor, educated or illiterate, clever or dull. Give him your heart and he will give you his."

My dog, Apollo, is so excited to see me when I get home that he makes me feel like a rock star meeting up with my number-one fan. Unconditional love is powerful. Laughing at a dog chasing its tail or a cat trying to pounce on a shadow is fun *and* good for you.

TEND A GARDEN. Growing plants can be deeply rewarding. Whether it's a field of greens or a couple of bonsai trees, gardening is one of the most common practices among the oldest-living people. Even keeping a collection of houseplants offers the benefit of adding oxygen and cleansing the air and may help your concentration.

EXPERIENCE FARM LIFE. Remember when I talked about breathing in phytoncides in nature? Farms offer a natural abundance of these beneficial bugs, and visiting working farms is one of my favorite pastimes. The Santa Ynez Valley in California—home to some of California's many olive groves—has become a special place for me. I jog in its vineyards, visit apple farms, ride horses, buy local olive oil, and meet up with friends for dinner, where we drink great wine. To me, this epitomizes the Wild Mediterranean way. Reconnecting with the land provides a terrific way to shake off the mental dust of a dreary or demanding day.

LAUGH. Do you remember the last time you really laughed? It felt good, right? Laughing out loud reduces stress hormones such as cortisol, and produces health-protecting hormones. I tape late-night talk shows and *Saturday Night Live* just to watch the opening monologue and laugh my you-know-what off, especially on days when I need a boost. Those cat videos that people share on Facebook? One university studied the effects of laughing at them and found they reduce feelings of anxiety and boost serotonin levels in the brain, which is the natural equivalent of popping a Xanax. So the next time you're caught watching one, just say, "It's medicinal!"

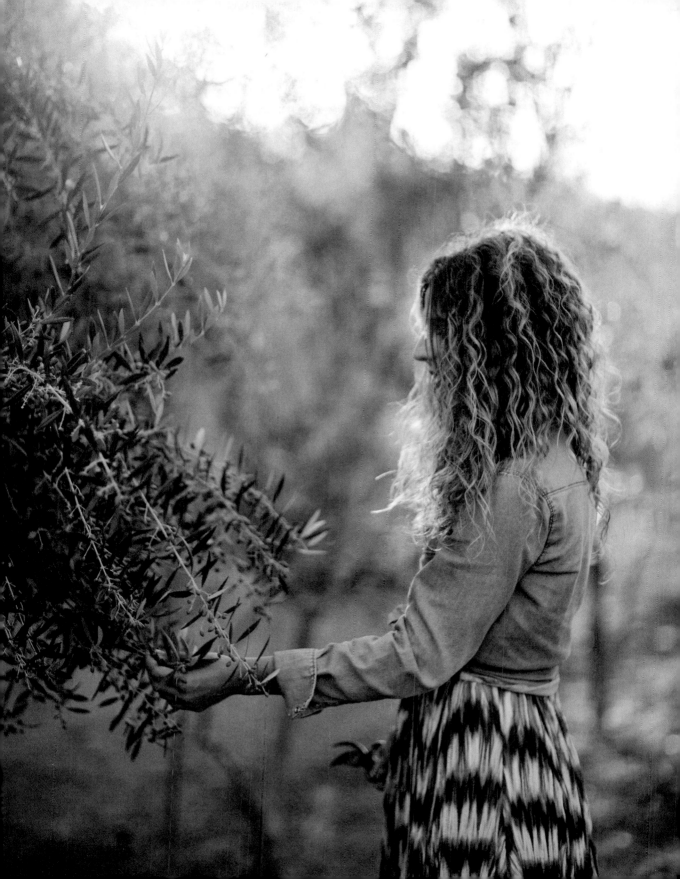

REDUCE STRESSFUL SCREEN TIME. Researchers found that looking at other people's seemingly perfect lives on Facebook can cause feelings of anxiety or inadequacy. Trust me, no one has a perfect life. Give yourself permission to unfriend or hide "friends" whose updates bug you. TV shows can cause stress, too, particularly the nightly news, crime shows, or all that pointless bickering on *Real Housewives*. Save your TV time for shows that educate, inspire, or make you laugh.

SAY "NO" TO GUILT. A common source of stress is taking on too much simply because saying "no" makes you feel guilty. But taking on too much is a common stress instigator, whether it's in your social or your professional life. Give yourself permission to determine your limits and learn to stick to them. Saying "no" to guilt also includes refusing to feel bad about what you eat. The beauty of the Wild Mediterranean lifestyle is that it accommodates—even demands—balance. Of course, you have to be honest with yourself as to whether you're truly doing your body a service with the foods you're feeding it, but stepping off the path now and then is not worth stressing over—consider it one more nice thing you can do for your gut!

AVOID TOXIC PEOPLE. Perhaps a friend pushes your buttons, or you feel routinely manipulated by a self-involved colleague. Some people are just a drag to be around. Toxic people are like the bad bacteria in our gut—you've got to strengthen your social immune system and kick them out of your life. There's a saying, "Letting people go is not an act of cruelty; it's an act of self-care." If you can't ditch someone from your life, then limit your time and exposure to that person to contain the damage. Spend more time with upbeat, active friends who make you feel good about yourself.

MANAGE YOUR TIME. Time is life's great equalizer. Everyone gets the same amount of hours each day. Randy Pausch, the famed Carnegie Mellon professor, said it best: "Being successful doesn't make you manage your time well. Managing your time well makes you successful." This applies to everything, from getting enough exercise and sleep to eating well to spending quality time with family and friends. Most Americans have a strong sense of "time poverty," and focus on having too few hours each day. Shift that perspective and instead focus on what's good enough or important enough to take up your precious time. What makes you happy to be alive? What gives your life a sense of purpose? Who do you truly want to spend your valuable hours with?

THE POWER OF SEX

Simply put, sex is not just a good time; it's great for your health. We humans are sexual creatures at our cores. Plus, sex is a great stress-busting exercise that burns between 75 to 150 calories per half hour, depending on how, um, robust your sessions tend to get.

Not only that, frequent sex may help you live longer. In a study published in the *British Medical Journal,* nine hundred generous men in the UK agreed to report the number of orgasms they had over a ten-year period. Those who averaged three or more orgasms a week had *half* the mortality rate of the others over the span of four years. Sex can aid your immune system and improve your mental prowess. People who have sex frequently tend to have a more positive outlook on life, and a stronger relationship with their partner. So, as the slogan goes, just do it!

ACCEPT WHAT YOU CANNOT CHANGE. Sometimes, we just have to deal. Put things in perspective. When you take a hard look at what's going on in the rest of the world, just how difficult are the challenges you are facing, really? In his amazing book *The Power of Now,* Eckhart Tolle states that there are three solutions to every problem: Accept it, change it, or leave it. If you can't accept it, change it. If you can't change it or leave it, accept it. Once you begin looking at life this way, you no longer feel the burden of attempting to fix what lies beyond your power.

BANISH BOREDOM. Surprisingly, a boring life can be stressful. Being bored is best described as feeling weary because you're unoccupied or lack interest in your current activity.

Unsurprisingly, boredom is perceived by your brain as negative, associating it with depression and aggression. Bored people, or those who don't engage in the things happening around themselves, often die younger than those who make an effort to feel energized most of the time.

Researchers discovered a connection between unhealthy eating, obesity, and boredom. What do you typically do when you're bored? Reach for a snack? Turn on the TV? Waste time online? In those moments, consider boredom a valuable signal. The next time you feel disengaged, make a list of things you've been meaning to do, such as hitting that museum exhibit you keep hearing about, going to a nursery to pick up a new houseplant, or even reorganizing your closet.

If you're bored at work, maybe it's time to consider a change, or to find a way to alter that job. I admire Jeff Bezos, the head of Amazon.com. Bezos believes most employees would be surprised to discover that their bosses want them to try new things to make a business better. Amazon's staff review process favors employees willing to try something new and fail, rather than those who play it safe. It goes back to the spaghetti test at the start of this chapter: "If you double the number of experiments you try in one year," Bezos says, "you double your potential for inventiveness." Want to be inspired? Watch *Shark Tank* and listen to how many people have developed their new businesses to get out of unsatisfying jobs.

PLAN FUN ACTIVITIES. People who work in the happiness business (think: Disney) know that anticipating something positive is a boon to our bliss quotient. Having something fun to look forward to helps us decompress from daily stress. Just anticipating a social event, or a vacation, or a play you have tickets for is so important; looking forward to it can make you as happy as the event itself.

Keep Calm and Sleep

The human microbiome is affected by sleep, although researchers aren't sure exactly how. They do know that disrupting your circadian rhythm—your body's internal time clock—can devastate a healthy gut. The resulting dysbiosis causes inflammation of the central nervous system. Your unsettled gut's microbes impact your sleep quality and how you react to stress in a complex set of "answer and call" interactions among the endocrine glands.

We spend one-third of our lives sleeping . . . or at least we should. It's easy to put off sleep. With much to do, it's tempting to burn the candle at both ends, but do so at your peril.

Getting enough sleep may be the single most important factor in predicting longevity, and is possibly more influential than diet, exercise, or your genes.

A lack of sleep also affects your weight. Sleep helps maintain a healthy balance of ghrelin, the hormone that make you feel hungry, and leptin, the hormone that makes you feel full. When you don't get enough sleep, your level of ghrelin goes up and your level of leptin goes down. This makes you feel hungrier than when you're well rested.

One of my clients, Brenda, is a beautiful, cheerful, and busy woman in her mid-sixties. She and her husband of thirty-five years travel extensively, both in the US and internationally. When she arrived in my office a few years ago, Brenda wasn't overweight, but she was interested in trimming down her body fat. "There's also something going on with my sleep," she said. "Something's not right."

In addition to her GI tests, I ordered a salivary panel. It showed her cortisol levels were totally off. When cortisol, a stress hormone, spikes, the body shifts into a "fight or flight" response, stimulating the sympathetic nervous system and adrenal glands. If the body remains in a state of constant stress, it burns out the adrenal system, strains the digestive tract, and causes cells to age more rapidly.

Cortisol levels should be at their highest in the morning to help you wake up and prepare to take on the day. They should be at their lowest at night, so you can wind down and sleep. Brenda's were almost the opposite.

I recommended that Brenda take an adaptogenic herb supplement (discussed in Chapter 2) to help balance, restore, and protect the body's systems. Adaptogenics are

> Your unsettled gut's microbes impact your sleep quality and how you react to stress in a complex set of "answer and call" interactions among the endocrine glands.

also particularly helpful in reducing and readjusting cortisol levels. I also had her monitoring her blood sugar levels to see if they were dipping too low at night (which could be remedied by having a bite of protein and fat). Turns out the Wild Mediterranean program is perfectly suited to support the adrenal glands and regulate blood sugar, which will in turn help you get a better night's sleep.

Create a Strong Social Network

We are social creatures. People with strong social networks tend to be healthier and live longer. In fact, the breadth of our social relationships may be one of best indicators of how long we'll live. The most social people, the ones with the most friends and acquaintances, live the longest. Being a loner, having a small circle of friends, or making social media your only pal can be as harmful to your health as smoking cigarettes, abusing alcohol, or being obese.

Having a strong sense of purpose can add years to your life, which is something I see first-hand when I go back to Greece. Everyone in the village, including the elderly, has a role and it's a factor in the impressive longevity of people who live on the island of Ikaria in Greece all the way to the inhabitants of Okinawa, home to the greatest number of centurions in the world.

ALCOHOL

Of course, part of socializing for many people involves clinking alcohol-filled glasses together in a friendly toast, right?

I'm not going to tell you to give up drinking. I'd be at odds with the approximately two billion people worldwide who drink alcohol on a daily basis. Instead, I want you to understand how alcohol affects your body so that you can make good decisions about what to drink, when and how much, and how to care for your biome afterwards.

When alcohol hits your system, your stomach emits an enzyme that turns alcohol into a chemical compound known as acetaldehyde. This compound, combined with the sugars from alcohol, creates inflammation throughout your body. While dehydration is often cited as the reason behind a hangover, it's really the impact of the acetaldehyde that causes your head to pound the morning after.

All alcohol stresses your microbiome and can contribute to dysbiosis and create a rift in your circadian rhythms, affecting your sleep. Remember what I said before about sleep and the microbiome? While the effect of alcohol on other parts of the body has been well documented, the study of alcohol's impact on the microbiome is still relatively new. Researchers have found that chronic alcohol consumption results in bacterial overgrowth in the small intestine (known as SIBO). Eating probiotic- and prebiotic-rich foods may help prevent or lessen the negative impact of alcohol on your gut.

Being generous can boost your health and lengthen your life, too. Generous people cope better when life throws them a curveball, such as a serious illness or the death of a family member. One year-long study logged the hours people spent helping others by running errands, doing housework or looking after their children. Those who spent the least time helping others were the most likely to suffer serious health problems or even die following a stressful situation.

You'll be glad to know that being social can strengthen your gut health, too. A study discovered chimps transfer bacterial colonies among themselves, helping to diversify their microbiomes. That same team plans to study humans to see if that's one of the reasons highly social people outlive wallflowers. So go out there and mingle. Your microbiome will thank you.

Moderate intake of wine with meals is part of the Wild Mediterranean way. Moderate means one glass of wine per day for women, or two for men. But hey, sometimes you want to celebrate, right? If you know you're going to have a big night out, you need to prep your gut. Here's how to lessen the negative impact of alcohol:

1) Pump up your water intake. Aim for at least three liters throughout the day before you drink.

2) Eat plenty of prebiotic as well as probiotic foods (see page 59). This will help prevent alcohol-induced dysbiosis.

3) Load up on vegetables the day before drinking and continue to make eating lots of vegetables a priority the day after. Coat them with extra-virgin olive oil or a little butter with sea salt. The day after a particularly indulgent evening is also a great time to start a pre-tox.

One remedy you should avoid completely, however, is a juice detox after a night of drinking. Since alcohol can contribute to SIBO, the last thing you want is more "sugar," healthy or not. And most juices are loaded with sugars owing to all the plants' fibers being stripped out. (Though, you could make your own juice in a high-power blender, which would give you a fiber-rich juice alternative.)

I find that wine is the best alcoholic beverage for the benefits it can provide, and recommend dry-farmed or biodynamic wines as your healthiest options. Although red wine is known for its polyphenols such as resveratrol, getting these from foods—such as pistachios, raspberries, and blueberries—is a better strategy than taking them in through alcohol. Fresh is always best.

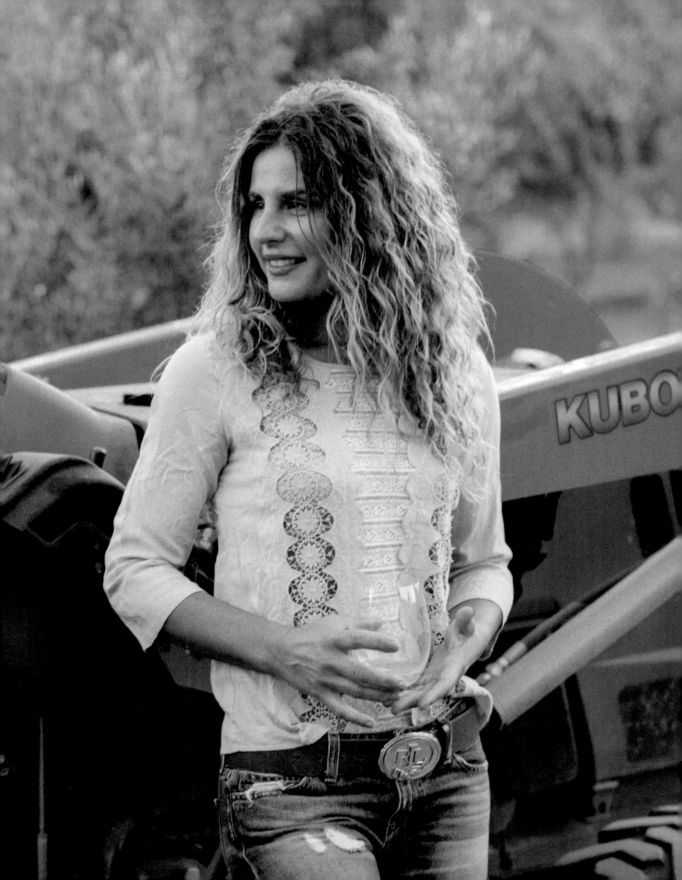

Get Wildly Beautiful

When I was about twenty years old, I visited a small seaside town in southern Italy. When I saw a fisherman walk by carrying a box of the most incredibly fresh and sweet-looking baby shrimp, I followed him into a nondescript seafood tavern. I got a seat looking out at the water, and next to me was a breathtakingly beautiful woman. She had perfect skin and gorgeous, shiny, thick black hair. She wore no makeup. I was studying nutrition at the time, so I of course observed what she ate—sardines, a platter of braised vegetables, and a glass of wine. We ended up chatting and I asked her about her lunch—was that what she usually ate? "This is what I was brought up on," she said. "We didn't have much money, so we ate whatever vegetables were fresh and a lot of fish." It was the first time I made the connection between diet and appearance. It makes sense: The better you eat, the better you look. That's the biggest beauty secret of Mediterranean women, and it's why following a Wild Mediterranean diet is more beneficial than any lotion or potion you could buy in the store.

That said, self-care is still an important part of life, which includes what we use on our skin. I'm not talking about beauty or self-care because of vanity. This part of your life is just as important as exercising and sleeping well, because your skin is your largest organ, and what you put on it enters the body and can affect your gut health. Making good choices about personal care products and cosmetics is important because many of them contain damaging chemicals.

Additives such as phthalates, parabens, triclosan, and oxybenzone can be found in everything from cosmetics to fragrance, hair products, soaps, and sunscreens; and animal studies show these chemicals interfere with the body's endocrine system, throwing our hormones out of balance. One study showed that even a short break from makeup, shampoos, and lotions with these chemicals can reduce the hormone disruption your body experiences.

The good news is that it's simple to create your own products with all-natural, inexpensive ingredients—and they work better than most of the expensive packaged stuff you can buy. Here are a few to get you started.

WILD MEDITERRANEAN SEA SPRAY

Bring the seaside to your everyday life. Thalassotherapy, or the therapeutic use of salt water, has been used in Mediterranean countries for hundreds of years. The idea is that you can get many of the benefits of the ocean by applying mineral-rich sea salt to your skin. Depending on the origin of the salt, it may contain sixty or more trace minerals, including copper, zinc, and iron. Formulated into a simple spray, you can absorb these minerals by applying it to the skin in the crook of your arms once or twice daily.

1 tablespoon Celtic sea salt

1 cup water

In a small pot, gently warm the salt and water. Allow the mixture to cool before transferring it to a glass apothecary spray mist bottle. Store at room temperature for up to 1 week or in the fridge for up to 1 month. Shake before using.

TUSCAN AROMATIC ROOM SPRAY

Sometimes one of the simplest ways to feel beautiful is to surround yourself with beautiful things. I'll never forget the aroma of Tuscany after a rainfall on one of my first trips to the gorgeous countryside. The scent of rich soil combined with the olives, wildflowers, and cypress trees was truly magical. When I got back home, I tried a few store-bought essential oil mixtures that were nice, but didn't really capture the heart of Tuscany. After tinkering a bit on my own, I managed to get as close as possible to bottling its essence. Here's a little piece of Tuscan rain and earth for your home.

½ cup spring water

20 drops cypress essential oil

10 drops eucalyptus essential oil

5 drops lemon essential oil

Combine all the ingredients in a 6-ounce glass spray bottle. Shake before each use.

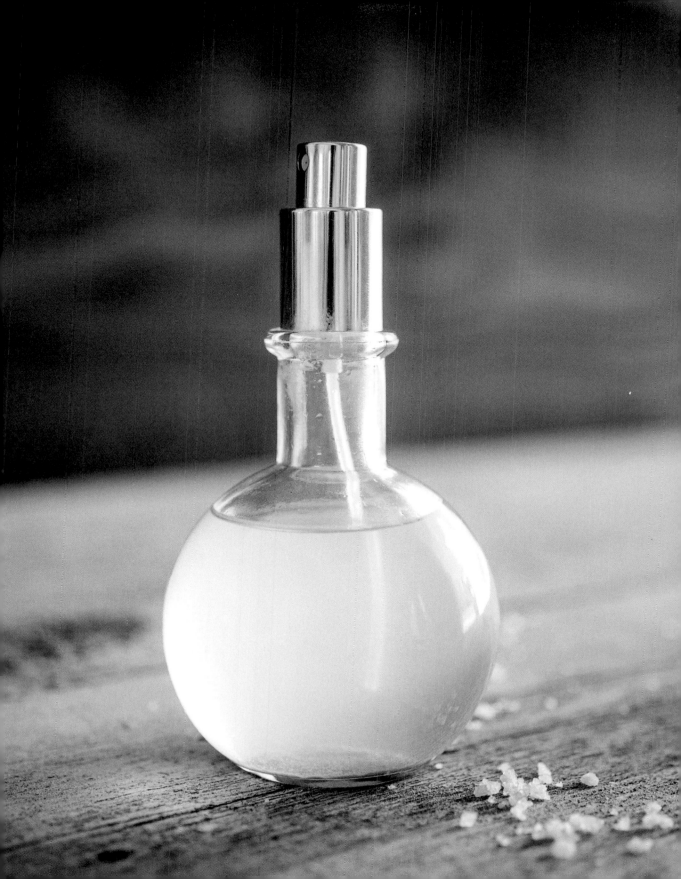

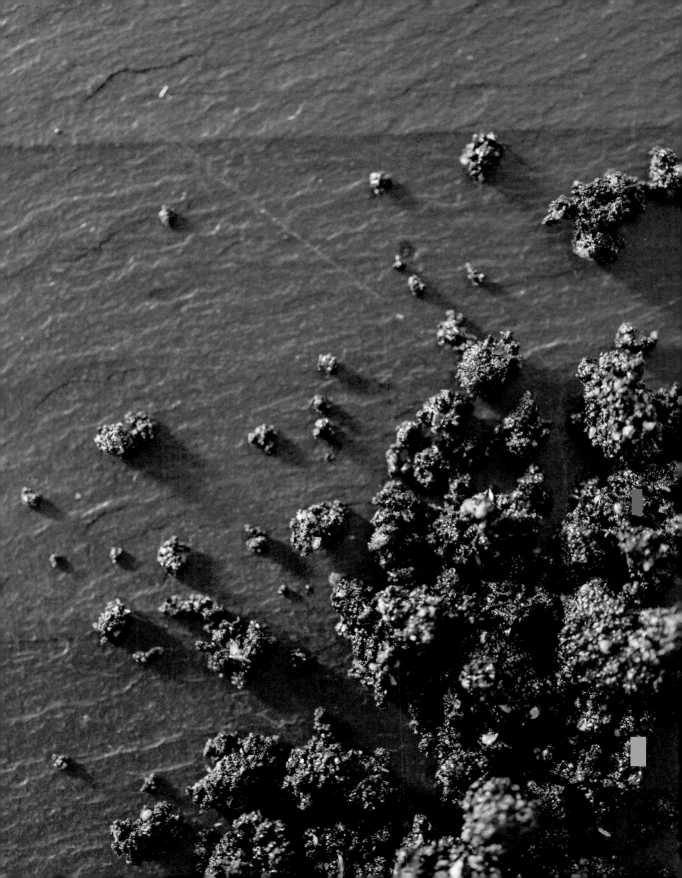

DRIED FIG AND COFFEE EXFOLIANT

The first time I made this recipe was in Palm Desert, California, and I used incredible local dates. Later I remembered that figs are a natural acne remedy and revised the formula to combine them with coffee, a natural exfoliant, and skin-conditioning coconut oil and olive oil. Here's the secret: Sit in the sun for 20 minutes and allow the mask to dry on your skin before rinsing it off. If you have an outside shower for rinsing, that's optimal, as the coffee can be messy. Or turn a garden hose on low and rinse off while you're still outside. If you shower inside, just be sure to rinse out your shower fully, so the coffee grounds don't stain your shower floor.

2 dried figs (stems removed)
¾ cup fine organic coffee grounds (used grounds are okay)
½ cup coconut oil
Extra-virgin olive oil, as needed

Add the figs, coffee grounds, and coconut oil to a high-powered blender and blend to make a paste. If the mixture is too thick, very slowly drizzle in a bit of olive oil until a smooth paste forms.

"HONEY, I'M HOT" EXFOLIANT

Exfoliating is essential for radiant skin and stimulating circulation. I recommend brushing your body daily with a dry loofah, and then using this blend for the face and neck (or on your derrière during bikini season). If you don't have almond meal in your cupboard, you can make it by grinding almonds to a coarse powder in a blender or food processor.

2 tablespoons organic, raw honey
1½ teaspoons baking soda
1 tablespoon almond meal

In a bowl, combine all the ingredients and stir to form a paste. Apply to the face, neck, and anywhere else you want to exfoliate. Scrub gently to remove dead, dull skin cells. Then allow it to sit on the skin: 10 minutes for the face and neck; 20 minutes for the body. Rinse thoroughly. Follow with moisturizer.

"OLIVE YOUR HAIR" SERUM

Mediterranean women have been treating their hair with olive oil for centuries, and it's my go-to conditioner. It keeps long, curly locks particularly shiny. Olive oil helps rejuvenate the hair follicles and moisturize the scalp, while the pumpkin soothes and deeply moisturizes, and the protein in the egg strengthens. Try this treatment once a week; it's great for both women and men.

½ cup extra-virgin olive oil

I tablespoon coconut oil

2 tablespoons pumpkin puree (canned organic is okay)

I egg yolk

In a small pot, combine the olive oil and coconut oil and warm gently. Remove from the heat and transfer to a small bowl. Stir in the pumpkin puree and egg yolk. Apply to the hair, wrap in a towel, and let sit for 1 hour. For best results, add heat from a blow dryer for 5 minutes every 20 minutes.

YIAYIA'S HORTA TONER

When you make Greek Wild Greens (page 113) or simple boiled greens, don't toss out the water! If you've used organic greens, the leftover braising liquid can do wonders for your skin topically as a natural polyphenol spritzer— or a natural antioxidant and protectant for the skin. What inspired me to make this toner was a similar product from a Palm Desert, California, shop called The Body Deli. I developed this version for my clients to use during their detox, especially if they were preparing for an important event, like a wedding, movie role, or even an appearance on the red carpet during awards season.

I cup braising liquid from cooking greens (page 113), cooled

I tablespoon apple cider vinegar

I teaspoon glycerin

Few drops of rosehip oil

In an apothecary glass spray bottle, combine the ingredients and place in refrigerator. Spritz directly onto your face and follow with your favorite moisturizer. Store in the refrigerator for up to 1 month.

CONCLUSION

WHEN I FIRST CAME UP WITH THE WILD MEDITERRANEAN CONCEPT, I DESCRIBED THIS REVOLUTIONary approach to health as "age-old, science-new." Returning to the rituals of simpler times armed with the knowledge of now is a potent combination for our wellness of body, mind, and spirit.

I've always known that immersing myself in the way of life practiced by my Greek relatives made me feel more vibrant and strong. I could see it in the mirror, too—the way spending just a month in their village would yield supple, sun-kissed skin; shiny, lustrous hair; and a lean, bloatless physique. It made sense: I was eating whole foods prepared at the peak of their seasonality (while not denying myself any essential macronutrients—hooray for healthy fats!), moving my body regularly and organically, connecting with nature on a daily basis, and participating in traditions that connected me with a sense of shared heritage. I was truly happy, inside and out.

So it came as no surprise that the newest frontiers of science validated the results that I'd observed empirically. Researchers have the ability to look at every nuance of our bodies in ways that were unimaginable ten years ago, connecting dots that have eluded the medical community for generations. Can all that data be overwhelming sometimes? Absolutely. But the beautiful thing is that all signs *aren't* pointing to taking the next miracle pill or undergoing newfangled surgical procedures when it comes to reclaiming our health. Quite the opposite. These findings tell us that we desperately need to get things back to basics.

The Wild Mediterranean lifestyle is composed of those basics. Innately, in stripping things down to their simplest practices—from what we eat to how we move to how we interact with others—we are benefitting our health at the deepest, most crucial level. Our bodies were not built to withstand the abuse of modern inventions, whether industrial farming practices and pesticide-soaked crops; or foods stuffed with additives, preservatives, and artificial coloring; or animals fed unnatural diets laced with hormones and antibiotics; or diets made up mostly of refined carbohydrates and little to no plants; or desk-oriented jobs that require long stretches of sitting (followed by hours vegging on the sofa); or isolation that comes from increasing dependence on technological communication; to almost complete separation from real, live nature. It's no wonder so many of us don't feel well!

And yet, people are beginning to realize this on their own. Take just five minutes to scroll through the social media outlet of your choice and you'll see no shortage of images of people reclaiming age-old practices. They're returning to the farm, returning to the kitchen, returning to tables shared with families and friends. They're saying no to processed food and yes to plants grown in their own communities (or backyards!); no to "timesavers" like microwaved meals and yes to simply (and quickly) prepared meals with a few quality ingredients; no to not knowing where their food is coming from, yes to digging in and getting their hands dirty (literally—hello, bacteria-rich soil) by growing their own. Whether it's in Omaha, Nebraska, or Los Angeles, California—that's the Wild Mediterranean way!

I know that making such lifestyle changes can seem daunting, especially if you're just beginning your Wild Mediterranean journey. I urge you to remember that with every small change you make, you're one step closer to feeling your best, with fewer chronic aches and pains, less digestive discomfort, less bloating, fewer skin complaints, no more lethargy. And because all of the recommendations in this book are meant to be carried with you for the rest of your life you won't find any suggestions that will make you feel deprived or joyless. On the contrary, this new approach to healthy living is meant to give you *more*—more foods to eat, more options for how to nourish your body and feel amazing, more opportunities to really connect with the outside world, and more ways to have fun and enjoy life. After all, science confirms that when we treat our bodies right, they give us back the most incredible gift: True health.

My website, stellametsovas.com, offers loads more advice and reassurance, plus even more delicious recipes. I also encourage you to connect with other people who are living the kind of life you're building for yourself. Embrace social media and use its powerful influence to help you as you go. Steep yourself in positive images and inspirational messaging. Engage with people who lift you up and share your outlook on how to live your best life.

And most important, give it up for yourself. Just by reading this book you've already started on your way to making significant, long-lasting changes that will profoundly better your life. Be sure to thank yourself for that—your body sure will.

Resources

Adaptogens

Positive Energy by YS Eco Bee Farms
https://www.amazon.com/
Positive-YS-Eco-Bee-Farms/dp/
B00028ND40?th=1

Raw Energy by Premier One
https://www.amazon.com/Energy
-Extreme-Premier-One-Caps/
dp/B0001VUJOK or http://
premieronenaturals.com/energy/
raw-energy-extreme.html

Bee Pollen / Royal Jelly

https://www.amazon.com/
YS-Organic-Bee-Propolis
-Capsules/dp/B000QS7HLG/
ref=lp_8086385011_1_16_a_it?srs
=8086385011&ie=UTF8&qid=14
78701611&sr=8-16

http://premieronenaturals.com/
royal-jelly-1000-1000mg-4.html

Food-Based Multivitamin

Whole Earth & Sea
http://www.wholeearthsea.com/
our-products/

New Chapter
http://www.newchapter.com/
vitamins

Garden of Life
https://www.gardenoflife.com/
content/product/why-choose
-vitamin-code/vitamin-code
-multivitamin-formulas/

Digestive

Gut-Pacs
www.gutpacs.com

Activated Charcoal

Source Naturals
https://www.amazon.com/
Source-Naturals-Charcoal
-Activated-Capsules/dp/
B00014CFKAI?th=1

Solaray
https://www.amazon.com/
Solaray-Activated-Charcoal
-Capsules-Count/dp/
B000TMM2V4

Botanic Choice
http://www.botanicchoice.com/
Digestive-Health/Charcoal
-Capsules-260-mg-60-capsules.axd

Prebiotics

Designs for Health
http://catalog.designsforhealth.
com/PaleoFiber-Powder-Unflavored

IsoThrive
https://www.isothrive.com

Prebiotin
https://www.prebiotin.com/
product-info/prebiotic-fiber/

Spirulina

HealthForce
https://healthforce.com/
superfoods-rejuvenation/
spirulina-manna

Nutrex-Hawaii
http://www.nutrex-hawaii.com/
hawaiian-spirulina-500mg-400
-tablets

Seaweed

Maine Coast
https://www.seaveg.com/shop/

Fish Oil

Carlson
http://www.carlsonlabs.com/p-107
-cod-liver-oil-lemon-flavor.aspx

Green Pasture
http://www.greenpasture.org/
public/Products/CodLiverOil/

MCT Oil

Now Foods
https://www.nowfoods.com/
sports-nutrition/mct-oil-liquid

Nature's Way
http://www.naturesway
.com/Product-Catalog/
Liquid-Coconut-Oil-10-oz

Cookware

All-Clad
http://www.all-clad.com/
Collections

Lodge Cast Iron
http://www.lodgemfg.com

Le Creuset
https://www.lecreuset.com

Romertopf
http://www.roemertopf.de/english/
produkte_roemertopf.htm

Olive Oil

The best domestic resource for olive oil is the **California Olive Council.**
https://www.cooc.com

California Olive Ranch
https://californiaoliveranch.com/
home-cooks/

Trader Joe's Premium 100% Greek Kalamata Extra Virgin Olive Oil
http://www.traderjoes.com/digin/
post/guide-to-evoo

Tassos
https://www.tassos.com/products/
tassos-olive-oils

Bone Broth
Kettle & Fire Grass-Fed Beef Bone Broth
https://www.kettleandfire.com

Pacific Foods Bone Broth
http://www.pacificfoods.com/food/
broths-stocks.aspx

Butter
Organic Valley
https://www.organicvalley.coop/
products/butter/

Meyenberg
http://meyenberg.com/
products-page/butter/
european-style-butter/

Kerrygold
http://kerrygoldusa.com

Eggs
Backyard Eggs by Vital Farms
http://vitalfarms.com/our-eggs/

The Happy Egg Co.
http://thehappyeggco.com

Sprouted Flour
Arrowhead Mills
http://www.arrowheadmills
.com/product/
organic-sprouted-wheat-flour

King Arthur
http://www.kingarthurflour.
com/shop/items/
organic-sprouted-wheat-flour-2-lb

Canned Tuna and Sardines
Wild Planet
http://www.wildplanetfoods.com/
our-products/

Yerba Mate
Eco Teas (Unsmoked)
http://yerbamate.com

Frozen fish
Sea to Table
http://www.sea2table.com

Meats
Pastured meats
http://www.eatwild.com/products/

Applegate Farms *Sausage
http://www.applegate.com/
products/dinner-sausage/category

Bread & Tortillas
Food For Life
http://www.foodforlife.com/
products?tid_1=All&tid=All

Coconut Vinegar
Thrive Market
https://thrivemarket.com/coconut
-secret-organic-raw-coconut-aminos

Wine
Dry Farm Wines
https://www.dryfarmwines.com

Beauty
Korres

100% Pure

Wedela

Burt's Bees

Dr. Hauschka

Dr. Bronner's

Acknowledgments

I'd like to thank my mother, Maria, who introduced me to the village and all its beauty. The summers in our *horio* inspired so much of what I'm doing today. Thank you for driving me to swim practice at 4:30 am; thank you for making me get right back on the horse after the first buck; thank you for making me the best fish soup.

To my literary agent, Chris Tomasino, thank you for your dedication and support throughout the entire journey. To my publisher, Pam Krauss, and the team at Pam Krauss Books and Avery—thank you!

To all my family and friends for your support. There are no words to describe the love and gratitude I have for you all! Thank you. Thank you . . .

I'm also extremely grateful to all my mentors and teachers along the way—you laid the groundwork for connecting the past to modern science.

To all my clients who were willing to explore the microbiome during a time when it might have been perceived as "experimental."

And finally, to Apollo, who's always inspired me throughout our time in nature.

Notes

Introduction: Why Wild Is Better

1   Burden of Gastrointestinal Disease in the United States: 2012 Update https://www.ncbi.nlm.nih.gov/pmc/articles/PMC3480553/

Chapter 1: Your Forgotten Organ

1   Center of Excellence for Nutritional Genomics (CENG) at the University of California, Davis http://nutrigenomics.ucdavis.edu

2   TLR Signaling in the Gut in Health and Disease http://www.jimmunol.org/content/174/8/4453.full

3   Robbins Pathologic Basis of Disease, 6e (Robbins Pathology) http://www.amazon.com/Robbins-Pathologic-Basis-Disease-Pathology/dp/072167335X (book reference)

4   Diet-Induced Dysbiosis of the Intestinal Microbiota and the Effects on Immunity and Disease https://www.ncbi.nlm.nih.gov/pmc/articles/PMC3448089/

5   The gut microbiome and the brain. https://www.ncbi.nlm.nih.gov/pubmed/25402818

6   The impact of microbiota on brain and behavior: mechanisms & therapeutic potential. https://www.ncbi.nlm.nih.gov/pubmed/24997043

7   The impact of microbiota on brain and behavior: mechanisms & therapeutic potential. https://www.ncbi.nlm.nih.gov/pubmed/24997043

8   The hot air and cold facts of dietary fibre https://www.ncbi.nlm.nih.gov/pmc/articles/PMC2659900/

9   Microbiota and diabetes: an evolving relationship http://gut.bmj.com/content/63/9/1513

10 Antibiotics Aren't Always the Answer https://www.cdc.gov/features/getsmart/

11 A healthy gastrointestinal microbiome is dependent on dietary diversity http://www.sciencedirect.com/science/article/pii/S2212877816000387

12 Mucosal healing in inflammatory bowel diseases: is there a place for nutritional supplementation? https://www.ncbi.nlm.nih.gov/pubmed/25208104

13 Prospective associations of vitamin D status with β-cell function, insulin sensitivity, and glycemia: the impact of parathyroid hormone status. https://www.ncbi.nlm.nih.gov/pubmed/24875346

14 Mammalian colonocytes possess a carrier-mediated mechanism for uptake of vitamin B3 (niacin): studies utilizing human and mouse colonic preparations. https://www.ncbi.nlm.nih.gov/pubmed/23744738

15 Dietary I(-) absorption: expression and regulation of the Na(+)/I(-) symporter in the intestine. https://www.ncbi.nlm.nih.gov/pubmed/25817864

16 Reshaping the gut microbiota: Impact of low calorie sweeteners and the link to insulin resistance? https://www.ncbi.nlm.nih.gov/pubmed/27090230

17 Weight influenced by microbes in the gut http://www.kcl.ac.uk/newsevents/news/newsrecords/2014/November/Weight-influenced-by-microbes-in-the-gut.aspx

18 Spatiotemporal maps reveal regional differences in the effects on gut motility for Lactobacillus reuteri and rhamnosus strains https://www.ncbi.nlm.nih.gov/pubmed/23316914

19 The Human Microbiome, Diet, and Health: Workshop Summary. https://www.ncbi.nlm.nih.gov/books/NBK154098/

20 Effects of Diurnal Variation of Gut Microbes and High-Fat Feeding on Host Circadian Clock Function and Metabolism http://www.cell.com/cell-host-microbe/abstract/S1931-3128(15)00123-7

21 The Gut Microbiota and their Metabolites: Potential Implications for the Host Epigenome. https://www.ncbi.nlm.nih.gov/pubmed/27161349

22 Influences of diet and the gut microbiome on epigenetic modulation in cancer and other diseases https://www.ncbi.nlm.nih.gov/pmc/articles/PMC4609101/

Chapter 2: The Wild Detox: Re-Wilding Your Body with Whole Foods

1   Evidence-based efficacy of adaptogens in fatigue, and molecular mechanisms related to their stress-protective activity. https://www.ncbi.nlm.nih.gov/pubmed/19500070

2   Pharmacotherapy of erectile dysfunction. https://www.ncbi.nlm.nih.gov/pubmed/16856460

3   Therapeutic potential of ginseng root preparations in treating diabetes mellitus. https://www.ncbi.nlm.nih.gov/pubmed/20095403

4   Too much folate in pregnant women increases risk for autism, study suggests https://www.sciencedaily.com/releases/2016/05/160511105352.htm

5   Associations of dietary folate, Vitamins B6 and

B12 and methionine intake with risk of breast cancer among African American and European American women. https://www.ncbi.nlm.nih.gov/pubmed/23996837

6 Effect of Royal Jelly on premenstrual syndrome among Iranian medical sciences students: a randomized, triple-blind, placebo-controlled study. https://www.ncbi.nlm.nih.gov/pubmed/25146061

7 The effect of royal jelly on oral mucositis in patients undergoing radiotherapy and chemotherapy. https://www.ncbi.nlm.nih.gov/pubmed/24919094

8 Lactobacillus kunkeei YB38 from honeybee products enhances IgA production in healthy adults. https://www.ncbi.nlm.nih.gov/pubmed/26121394

9 Royal Jelly and its dual role in TNBS colitis in mice. https://www.ncbi.nlm.nih.gov/pubmed/25821860

10 Mechanisms of the Effects of Probiotics on Symbiotic Digestion. https://www.ncbi.nlm.nih.gov/pubmed/26638234

11 Prebiotic consumption and the incidence of overweight in a Mediterranean cohort: the Seguimiento Universidad de Navarra Project. https://www.ncbi.nlm.nih.gov/pubmed/26561624

12 Optimization of the treatment of the patients presenting with chronic venous insufficiency in the lower extremities with the use of the modern methods of thalassotherapy. https://www.ncbi.nlm.nih.gov/pubmed/24437203

13 The influence of different types of bathes for general health on the efficiency of combined spa and resort treatment of coronary heart disease. https://www.ncbi.nlm.nih.gov/pubmed/21988021

14 Intestinal Short Chain Fatty Acids and their Link with Diet and Human Health https://www.ncbi.nlm.nih.gov/pmc/articles/PMC4756104/

15 Review article: dietary fibre–microbiota interactions https://www.ncbi.nlm.nih.gov/pmc/articles/PMC4949558/

16 Roles for vitamin K beyond coagulation. https://www.ncbi.nlm.nih.gov/pubmed/19400704

17 Carotenoid bioavailability is higher from salads ingested with full-fat than with fat-reduced salad dressings as measured with electrochemical detection. http://ajcn.nutrition.org/content/80/2/396.full

18 Glucosinolates and isothiocyanates in health and disease. https://www.ncbi.nlm.nih.gov/pubmed/22578879

19 Digestibility and prebiotic properties of potato rhamnogalacturonan I polysaccharide and its galactose-rich oligosaccharides/oligomers. https://www.ncbi.nlm.nih.gov/pubmed/26572449

20 Anthocyanins as inflammatory modulators and the role of the gut microbiota. https://www.ncbi.nlm.nih.gov/pubmed/27260462

21 Old Things New View: Ascorbic Acid Protects the Brain in Neurodegenerative Disorders https://www.ncbi.nlm.nih.gov/pubmed/26633354

22 Effects of almond and pistachio consumption on gut microbiota composition in a randomised cross-over human feeding study. https://www.ncbi.nlm.nih.gov/pubmed/24642201

23 Mucosal healing in inflammatory bowel diseases: is there a place for nutritional supplementation? https://www.ncbi.nlm.nih.gov/pubmed/25208104

24 Vitamin B_{12} as a modulator of gut microbial ecology. https://www.ncbi.nlm.nih.gov/pubmed/25440056

25 Nutrition meets the microbiome: micronutrients and the microbiota http://onlinelibrary.wiley.com/doi/10.1111/nyas.13145/abstract

26 Prospective associations of vitamin D status with β-cell function, insulin sensitivity, and glycemia: the impact of parathyroid hormone status. https://www.ncbi.nlm.nih.gov/pubmed/24875346

27 Influence of dietary fat on intestinal microbes, inflammation, barrier function and metabolic outcomes. https://www.ncbi.nlm.nih.gov/pubmed/24355793

28 Mammalian colonocytes possess a carrier-mediated mechanism for uptake of vitamin B3 (niacin): studies utilizing human and mouse colonic preparations. https://www.ncbi.nlm.nih.gov/pubmed/23744738

29 Bacteria as vitamin suppliers to their host: a gut microbiota perspective. https://www.ncbi.nlm.nih.gov/pubmed/22940212

30 Mammalian colonocytes possess a carrier-mediated mechanism for uptake of vitamin B3 (niacin): studies utilizing human and mouse colonic preparations. https://www.ncbi.nlm.nih.gov/pubmed/23744738

31 Proteins and Carbohydrates from Red Seaweeds: Evidence for Beneficial Effects on Gut Function and Microbiota. https://www.ncbi.nlm.nih.gov/pubmed/26308006

32 Seaweed-rich diet leaves its mark on gut microbes. http://www.nature.com/news/2010/100407/full/news.2010.169.html

33 The therapeutic management of gut barrier leaking: the emerging role for mucosal barrier protectors. https://www.ncbi.nlm.nih.gov/pubmed/25855934

34 Green vegetables directly influence immune defences and help maintain intestinal health http://dx.doi.org/10.1016/j.cell.2011.09.025

35 Protection of humans by plant glucosinolates:

efficiency of conversion of glucosinolates to isothiocyanates by the gastrointestinal microflora. https://www.ncbi.nlm.nih.gov/pubmed/22318753

36   A study of the effect of dietary fiber fractions obtained from artichoke (Cynara cardunculus L. var. scolymus) on the growth of intestinal bacteria associated with health. https://www.ncbi.nlm.nih.gov/pubmed/25904284

37   Effects of chlorophyll and chlorophyllin on low-dose aflatoxin B(1) pharmacokinetics in human volunteers. https://www.ncbi.nlm.nih.gov/pubmed/19952359

38   Annual Fasting; the Early Calories Restriction for Cancer Prevention https://www.ncbi.nlm.nih.gov/pmc/articles/PMC3648937/

39   Screening of a Marine Algal Extract for Antifungal Activities. https://www.ncbi.nlm.nih.gov/pubmed/26108521

40   Marine polysaccharides from algae with potential biomedical applications. https://www.ncbi.nlm.nih.gov/pubmed/25988519

41   Proteins and Carbohydrates from Red Seaweeds: Evidence for Beneficial Effects on Gut Function and Microbiota. https://www.ncbi.nlm.nih.gov/pubmed/26308006

42   Dietary medium-chain triacylglycerols suppress accumulation of body fat in a double-blind, controlled trial in healthy men and women. https://www.ncbi.nlm.nih.gov/pubmed/11694608

43   Fatty acids, lipid emulsions and the immune and inflammatory systems. https://www.ncbi.nlm.nih.gov/pubmed/25471799

Chapter 3: The Wild Kitchen

1   Glyphosate's Suppression of Cytochrome P450 Enzymes and Amino Acid Biosynthesis by the Gut Microbiome: Pathways to Modern Diseases. http://www.mdpi.com/1099-4300/15/4/1416

2   Vitamin Retention in Eight Fruits and Vegetables: A Comparison of Refrigerated and Frozen Storage http://www.frozenfoodfacts.org/research/new-study-reinforces-nutritional-benefits-frozen-fruits-and-vegetables

3   High polyphenol, low probiotic diet for weight loss because of intestinal microbiota interaction. https://www.ncbi.nlm.nih.gov/pubmed/20955691

4   Potential of rosemary oil to be used in drug-resistant infections. https://www.ncbi.nlm.nih.gov/pubmed/17900043

5   Apigenin and Breast Cancers: From Chemistry to Medicine. https://www.ncbi.nlm.nih.gov/pubmed/25738871

6   Fish consumption and the 30-year risk of fatal myocardial infarction. http://www.nejm.org/doi/pdf/10.1056/NEJM199704103361502

7   The Role of Microbial Amino Acid Metabolism in Host Metabolism https://www.ncbi.nlm.nih.gov/pmc/articles/PMC4425181/

8   Ensuring Modern, Timely Decisions for Infrastructure Projects http://blogs.usda.gov/2013/05/17/

9   Good Seafood Guide http://www.ewg.org/research/ewgs-good-seafood-guide

10   Glyphosate, pathways to modern diseases II: Celiac sprue and gluten intolerance. https://www.ncbi.nlm.nih.gov/pubmed/24678255

11   Glyphosate is a probably human carcinogen. https://monographs.iarc.fr/ENG/Monographs/vol112/mono112-09.pdf

12   Glyphosate, pathways to modern diseases II: Celiac sprue and gluten intolerance. https://www.ncbi.nlm.nih.gov/pmc/articles/PMC3945755/

13   Obesity threatens to cut U.S. life expectancy, new analysis suggests. https://www.nia.nih.gov/newsroom/2005/03/obesity-threatens-cut-u-s-life-expectancy-new-analysis-suggests

14   Lactose intolerance: https://ghr.nlm.nih.gov/condition/lactose-intolerance

15   Oligosaccharides isolated from goat milk reduce intestinal inflammation in a rat model of dextran sodium sulfate-induced colitis. https://www.ncbi.nlm.nih.gov/pubmed/16375993

16   Anti-inflammatory and anti-allergic properties of donkey's and goat's milk. https://www.ncbi.nlm.nih.gov/pubmed/24450455

17   The 2-monoacylglycerol moiety of dietary fat appears to be responsible for the fat-induced release of GLP-1 in humans. https://www.ncbi.nlm.nih.gov/pubmed/26178726

18   Health effects of olive oil polyphenols: recent advances and possibilities for the use of health claims. https://www.ncbi.nlm.nih.gov/pubmed/23450515

19   A food bank proves a healthy Mediterranean diet is cheaper than a junky American one. https://www.fastcoexist.com/3055157/a-food-bank-proves-a-healthy-mediterranean-diet-is-cheaper-than-a-junky-american-one

20   Wine consumption and intestinal redox homeostasis. https://www.ncbi.nlm.nih.gov/pubmed/25009781

21   In vitro bioconversion of polyphenols from black tea and red wine/grape juice by human intestinal microbiota displays strong interindividual variability. https://www.ncbi.nlm.nih.gov/pubmed/20726519

22   Wine consumption and intestinal redox homeostasis. https://www.ncbi.nlm.nih.gov/pubmed/25009781
23   Ibid.

Chapter 4: Village-To-Table Recipes

1   Reduction in dietary diversity impacts richness of human gut microbiota. https://www.sciencedaily.com/releases/2016/03/160315104210.htm
2   Libyan Thymus capitatus essential oil: antioxidant, antimicrobial, cytotoxic and colon pathogen adhesion-inhibition properties. https://www.ncbi.nlm.nih.gov/pubmed/26033505
3   The intestinal microbiome and skeletal fitness: Connecting bugs and bones. https://www.ncbi.nlm.nih.gov/pubmed/25840106
4   Inhibitory effect of maple syrup on the cell growth and invasion of human colorectal cancer cells. https://www.ncbi.nlm.nih.gov/pubmed/25647359
5   Ibid.
6   High polyphenol, low probiotic diet for weight loss because of intestinal microbiota interaction. https://www.ncbi.nlm.nih.gov/pubmed/20955691
7   The impact of dietary fibers on dendritic cell responses in vitro is dependent on the differential effects of the fibers on intestinal epithelial cells. https://www.ncbi.nlm.nih.gov/pubmed/25620425
8   Jerusalem artichoke and chicory inulin in bakery products affect faecal microbiota of healthy volunteers. https://www.ncbi.nlm.nih.gov/pubmed/17445348
9   Effects of almond and pistachio consumption on gut microbiota composition in a randomised cross-over human feeding study. https://www.ncbi.nlm.nih.gov/pubmed/24642201
10 The screening method of a bifidogenic dietary fiber extracted from inedible parts of vegetables. https://www.ncbi.nlm.nih.gov/pubmed/19763042
11 The ageing gastrointestinal tract. https://www.ncbi.nlm.nih.gov/pubmed/26560524
12 Ta chòrta: wild edible greens used in the Graecanic area in Calabria, Southern Italy. https://www.ncbi.nlm.nih.gov/pubmed/16843569
13 Resistant Starch Alters the Microbiota-Gut Brain Axis: Implications for Dietary Modulation of Behavior. https://www.ncbi.nlm.nih.gov/pubmed/26745269
14 Human gut flora-fermented nondigestible fraction from cooked bean (Phaseolus vulgaris L.) modifies protein expression associated with apoptosis, cell cycle arrest, and proliferation in human adenocarcinoma colon cancer cells. https://www.ncbi.nlm.nih.gov/pubmed/23194196

15 Nutritional aspects of depression. https://www.ncbi.nlm.nih.gov/pubmed/26402520
16 Environmental influences on T regulatory cells in inflammatory bowel disease. https://www.ncbi.nlm.nih.gov/pubmed/21295492
17 Mushrooms and Health Summit proceedings. https://www.ncbi.nlm.nih.gov/pubmed/24812070
18 Gut microbiome in health and disease: Linking the microbiome-gut-brain axis and environmental factors in the pathogenesis of systemic and neurodegenerative diseases. https://www.ncbi.nlm.nih.gov/pubmed/26627987
19 Chicory extract's influence on gut bacteria of abdominal obesity rat. https://www.ncbi.nlm.nih.gov/pubmed/25272847
20 The therapeutic management of gut barrier leaking: the emerging role for mucosal barrier protectors. https://www.ncbi.nlm.nih.gov/pubmed/25855934
21 Effect of garlic powder on the growth of commensal bacteria from the gastrointestinal tract. https://www.ncbi.nlm.nih.gov/pubmed/22480662
22 Metabolomics view on gut microbiome modulation by polyphenol-rich foods. https://www.ncbi.nlm.nih.gov/pubmed/22905879

Chapter 5: How to Live Wild

1   The Gastrointestinal Circulation https://www.ncbi.nlm.nih.gov/books/NBK53092/
2   Ibid.
3   Get Up. Get Out. Don't Sit. http://well.blogs.nytimes.com/2012/10/17/get-up-get-out-dont-sit/
4   Owning a dog may help you live longer, happier: study http://www.news.com.au/lifestyle/health/owning-a-dog-may-help-you-live-longer-happier-study/news-story/b12a490b2eee1991ab9a1a36ec8b88f2
5   A dog could be your heart's best friend http://www.health.harvard.edu/blog/a-dog-could-be-your-hearts-best-friend-201305226291
6   Benefits of indoor plants on attention capacity in an office setting. http://www.sciencedirect.com/science/article/pii/S0272494410001027
7   Selecting the right house plant could improve indoor air. https://www.acs.org/content/acs/en/pressroom/newsreleases/2016/august/selecting-the-right-house-plant-could-improve-indoor-air-animation.html
8   Anticipating A Laugh Reduces Our Stress Hormones, Study Shows. https://www.sciencedaily.com/releases/2008/04/080407114617.htm
9   Not-so-guilty pleasure: Viewing cat videos boosts energy and positive emotions, IU study finds. http://

news.indiana.edu/releases/iu/2015/06/internet-cat
-video-research.shtml

10 Negative social comparison on Facebook and
    depressive symptoms: Rumination as a mechanism.
    Psychology of Popular Media Culture, 2, 161–170.
    Feinstein, B.A., Herschenberg, R., Bhatia, V., Latack,
    J. A., Meuwly, N., & Davila, J. (2013).

11 Boredom, sustained attention and the default
    mode network. https://www.ncbi.nlm.nih.gov/
    pubmed/26979438

12 Bored to death? https://academic.oup.com/ije/
    article/39/2/370/684049/Bored-to-death

13 Boredom proneness and emotion regulation predict
    emotional eating http://journals.sagepub.com/doi/
    abs/10.1177/1359105315573439

14 How to design happiness. https://www
    .fastcodesign.com/3058237/innovation-by-design/
    how-to-design-happiness

15 Sex and death: are they related? Findings from the
    Caerphilly cohort study. http://www.bmj.com/
    content/315/7123/1641

16 All About Sex. https://www.psychologytoday.com/
    blog/all-about-sex

17 Human Gut Bacteria Are Sensitive to Melatonin and
    Express Endogenous Circadian Rhythmicity. https://
    www.ncbi.nlm.nih.gov/pubmed/26751389

18 The gut microbiome and the brain. https://www.ncbi
    .nlm.nih.gov/pubmed/25402818

19 The promise of sleep: A pioneer in sleep medicine
    explores the vital connection between health,
    happiness, and a good night's sleep. http://psycnet.apa
    .org/psycinfo/2000–07284–000

20 Why Is Sleep Important? https://www.nhlbi.nih.gov/
    health/health-topics/topics/sdd/why

21 Social Relationships and Mortality Risk: A Meta-
    analytic Review. http://journals.plos.org/plosmedicine/
    article?id=10.1371/journal.pmed.1000316

22 Ibid.

23 Ibid.

24 Doing for Others Also Benefits Health of Altruistic
    https://psychcentral.com/news/2013/02/06/doing
    -for-others-also-benefits-health-of-altruistic/51274
    .html

25 Ibid.

26 Social behavior shapes the chimpanzee pan-
    microbiome. http://advances.sciencemag.org/
    content/2/1/e1500997

27 The Gastrointestinal Microbiome: Alcohol Effects on
    the Composition of Intestinal Microbiota https://www
    .arcr.niaaa.nih.gov/arcr372/article07.htm

28 Teen girls see big drop in chemical exposure with
    switch in cosmetics. https://www.sciencedaily.com/
    releases/2016/03/160307113720.htm

29 Effect of hydrothermal processing on total
    polyphenolics and antioxidant potential of
    underutilized leafy vegetables, Boerhaavia diffusa and
    Portulaca oleracea. https://www.ncbi.nlm.nih.gov/
    pmc/articles/PMC4025293/

Index

Page numbers in *italics* refer to photos.

A

Avgolemono Sauce, 142, 145

B

baked beans, 121–23
Baklava Butter, *180*, 181
basic recipes
    Fish Stock, 175
    Mineral-Rich Bone Broth, 176
    Mom's Secret Tzatziki, 177
    Roasted Vegetable Stock, 174
    Wild Vinaigrette, 173
Basque-Style Cod, 167
beans and legumes
    Beans: Four Countries, Four Ways, 121–23
    Fava with Roasted Vegetables, *124*, 125–26
    French-Meets-Greek Salad, 104
    Jackson Pollock's Paella, *132*, 133–34
    Myconian-Inspired Black-Eyed Peas, 128, *129*
    processed soy, 43
    St. Barts–Style Chilled Pea Soup, 112
beauty products. *See* personal care products
beef
    Braised Meat: Four Countries, Four Ways, 161–63
    Burger with Whipped Potatoes, *152*, 153
    California-Style Homemade Gyro with Sprouted
        Tortilla and Tzatziki, 139
    From-the-Village Stuffed Zucchini, *140*, 141–42
    Herb-Scented Meatballs, 146–47
    Mineral-Rich Bone Broth, 176
    Moussaka, 150–51
    in pre-tox meal plan, 57
berries
    Berry and Chicken Salad, 73
    Chocolate Yogurt Sundae, 179
    in detox, 55
    Sprouted "Crepes," 97
beverages
    alcoholic drinks, 198–99
    caffeine in, 50
    Lavender Lemonade Tonic, 73

    Peppermint and Chamomile Tea, 73
    in Wild Mediterranean diet, 89–90
Black-Eyed Peas, Myconian-Inspired, 128, *129*
Bone Broth, Mineral-Rich, 176
Braised Chicken Thighs from Avignon, 148, *149*
Braised Meat: Four Countries, Four Ways,
    161–63
Braised Turkey Breast, 154–55
breakfasts
    Deep-Dish Frittata, 95
    Sprouted Cinnamon-Maple French Toast, 99
    Sprouted "Crepes," 97
    Yiayia's Eggs Mati, 96
Briam, *114*, 115–16
broths and stocks
    in detox, 58–59
    Fish Stock, 175
    Mineral-Rich Bone Broth, 176
    Roasted Vegetable Stock, 174
Burger with Whipped Potatoes, *152*, 153
Butternut Squash and Basil, Rigatoni with,
    130–31

C

California-Style Homemade Gyro with Sprouted
    Tortilla and Tzatziki, 139
Carrot and Cabbage Kraut, 59
Catalan Gazpacho, 109
cheese
    Burger with Whipped Potatoes, *152*, 153
    Endive Salad from Beaune, 102, *103*
    French-Meets-Greek Salad, 104
    Greek-Style Baked Beans, 122
    Myconian-Inspired Black-Eyed Peas, 128, *129*
    Not-Your-Typical Greek Salad, 110, *111*
    Pizza à la Stella, 137
    Risotto Classico, 136
    "Root-Down" Salad, *106*, 107
    Spinach Pie with Sprouted Wheat Crust,
        118–19
    Sprouted "Crepes," 97

chicken
  Berry and Chicken Salad, 73
  Braised Chicken Thighs from Avignon, 148, *149*
  California-Style Homemade Gyro with Sprouted
      Tortilla and Tzatziki, 139
  in detox, 58
  Greek-Style Lemon Chicken, 75
  Italian-Style Turkey 'n' Onion Soup (chicken
      option), 74
  Jackson Pollock's Paella, *132*, 133–34
  Mineral-Rich Bone Broth, 176
  to poach or grill, 58
  Roast Chicken: Four Countries, Four Ways, *156*,
      157–58
  rubs for, 158
  sausage, *in* Jackson Pollock's Paella, *132*, 133–34
  sausage, *in* Spanish-Style Baked Beans, 122
  Stuffed Sweet Potato, 74
Chilled Pea Soup, St. Barts–Style, 112
Chips, Sunchoke, 108
Chocolate Yogurt Sundae, 179
Cod, Basque-Style, 167
"Crepes," Sprouted, 97

D
dairy foods, 86–87. *See also* cheese; yogurt
Deep-Dish Frittata, 95
desserts
  Baklava Butter, *180*, 181
  Chocolate Yogurt Sundae, 179
detox
  caffeine during, 50
  diagnostic tests, 51–53
  foods for, 43–45, 54–61
  meal guidelines, 63–64
  purpose of, 40
  recipes, 73–75
  sample regimen, 65
  to schedule, 42–43
  supplements, 45–49
  tips for success, 71
  See also land-tox/sea-tox; pre-tox; Wild Detox
diet. *See* Wild Mediterranean diet
digestive health. *See* gut microbiome and digestive
    health
Dill Baked Salmon, 75
Dried Fig and Coffee Exfoliant, 205

drinks
  alcoholic drinks, 198–99
  caffeine in, 50
  Lavender Lemonade Tonic, 73
  Peppermint and Chamomile Tea, 73
  in Wild Mediterranean diet, 89–90

E
eggs
  Deep-Dish Frittata, 95
  Not-Your-Typical Greek Salad, 110, *111*
  Yiayia's Eggs Mati, 96
Endive Salad from Beaune, 102, *103*
Everyone's Fish Stew, *168*, 169
exercise, 77, 185–89
exfoliants
  Dried Fig and Coffee Exfoliant, 205
  "Honey, I'm Hot" Exfoliant, 205

F
Fava with Roasted Vegetables, *124*, 125–26
fermented foods
  Carrot and Cabbage Kraut, 59
  dairy products, 86–87
  in detox, 59
  as probiotics, 47
fish and shellfish
  in detox, 57
  Dill Baked Salmon, 75
  Everyone's Fish Stew, *168*, 169
  Fish in Parchment: Four Countries, Four Ways,
      166–67
  Fish Stock, 175
  Italian-Style Bean Salad, 123
  Jackson Pollock's Paella, *132*, 133–34
  Lemony Fish Wrapped in Grapes Leaves, 165
  mercury and sustainability concerns, 85–86
  to sauté, 57
  Sweet Scallop Skewers, 170, *171*
French-Meets-Greek Salad, 104
French-Style Baked Beans, 123
French-Style Braised Beef, 163
French Toast, Sprouted Cinnamon-Maple, 99
Fresh Salad, 73
Fricassee, *144*, 145
Frittata, Deep-Dish, 95
From-the-Village Stuffed Zucchini, *140*, 141–42

fruits
    Berry and Chicken Salad, 73
    Chocolate Yogurt Sundae, 179
    in detox, 55
    Endive Salad from Beaune, 102, *103*
    Myconian-Inspired Black-Eyed Peas, 128, *129*
    options, 80, 81
    Sprouted "Crepes," 97

G
Gazpacho, Catalan, 109
grains
    Braised Chicken Thighs from Avignon, 148, *149*
    California-Style Homemade Gyro with Sprouted
        Tortilla and Tzatziki, 139
    From-the-Village Stuffed Zucchini, *140*, 141–42
    Herb-Scented Meatballs, 146–47
    Jackson Pollock's Paella, *132*, 133–34
    Not-Your-Typical Greek Salad, 110, *111*
    oats, in detox, 61
    Pizza à la Stella, 137
    processed and refined, 43, 82–83
    Rigatoni with Butternut Squash and Basil, 130–31
    Risotto Classico, 136
    Spinach Pie with Sprouted Wheat Crust, 118–19
    Sprouted Cinnamon-Maple French Toast, 99
    Sprouted "Crepes," 97
    wheat intolerance, 82–83
Grape Leaves, Lemony Fish Wrapped in, 165
Greek Salad, Not-Your-Typical, 110, *111*
Greek-Style Baked Beans, 122
Greek-Style Braised Beef, 162
Greek-Style Lemon Chicken, 75
Greek-Style Rub, 158
Greek-Style Sea Bass, 167
Greek Wild Greens with Olive Oil and Lemon, 113
greens
    Berry and Chicken Salad, 73
    Burger with Whipped Potatoes, *152*, 153
    Carrot and Cabbage Kraut, 59
    in detox, 54–55, 59–60, 61
    Endive Salad from Beaune, 102, *103*
    French-Meets-Greek Salad, 104
    Fresh Salad, 73
    Fricassee, *144*, 145
    Greek Wild Greens with Olive Oil and Lemon, 113
    Italian-Style Bean Salad, 123

    Lucca-Style Salad, 105
    Rustic Vegetable Soup, 75
    Spanish-Style Baked Beans, 122
    Spinach Pie with Sprouted Wheat Crust, 118–19
    Stuffed Sweet Potato, 74
gut microbiome and digestive health
    benefit of Mediterranean foods and lifestyle,
        20–22, 27
    dysbiosis and associated health disorders, 20, 27,
        29–31, 32, 35
    exercise, 183–84
    immune system, 28–29
    prebiotic and probiotic foods, 47, 48, 59, 60–61
    to restore balance, 32–34
    stress management, 184
    tests and analyses, 31, 51–53
    weight control, 35–36
Gyro with Sprouted Tortilla and Tzatziki, California-
    Style Homemade, 139

H
Herb-Scented Meatballs, 146–47
"Honey, I'm Hot" Exfoliant, 205

I
Italian-Inspired Rub, 158
Italian-Style Bean Salad, 123
Italian-Style Braised Beef, 162
Italian-Style Salmon, 167
Italian-Style Turkey 'n' Onion Soup, 74

J
Jackson Pollock's Paella, *132*, 133–34

K
Kraut, Carrot and Cabbage, 59

L
lamb
    California-Style Homemade Gyro with Sprouted
        Tortilla and Tzatziki, 139
    Fricassee, *144*, 145
    From-the-Village Stuffed Zucchini, *140*, 141–42
    Herb-Scented Meatballs, 146–47
    Mineral-Rich Bone Broth, 176
    Moussaka, 150–51
land-based main dishes. *See* beef; chicken; lamb; turkey

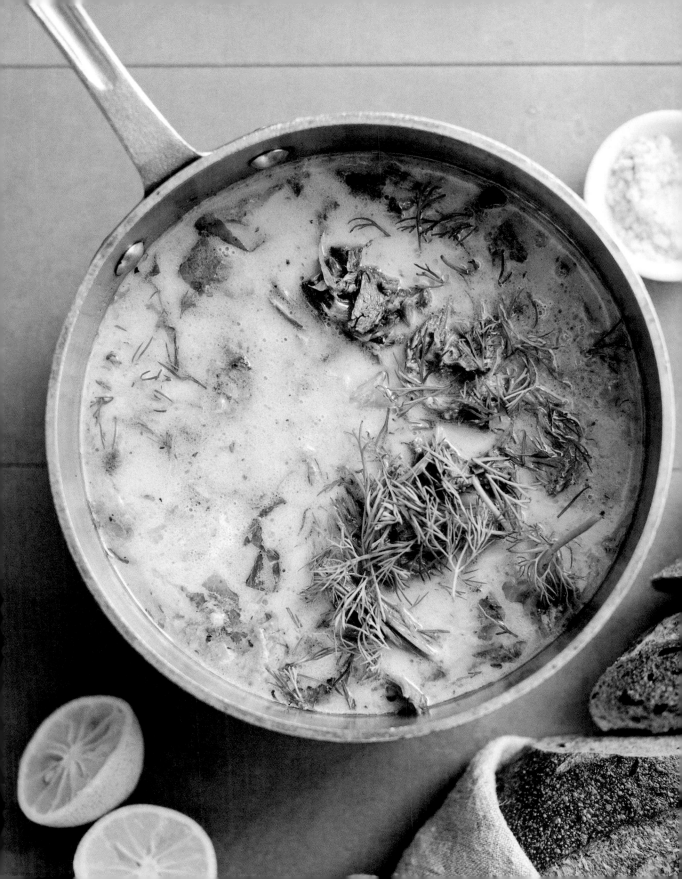

land-tox/sea-tox
    customization for specific needs, 34, 40, 67
    foods for, 54–60
    intermittent fasting, 66
    sample regimen, 69
    supplements, 68
Lavender Lemonade Tonic, 73
legumes. *See* beans and legumes
Lemon Chicken, Greek-Style, 75
Lemony Fish Wrapped in Grapes Leaves, 165
lifestyle. *See* Wild Mediterranean lifestyle
Lucca-Style Salad, 105

M
main dishes from the land. *See* beef; chicken; lamb;
    turkey
main dishes from the sea. *See* fish and shellfish
meat and poultry. *See also* beef; chicken; lamb;
    turkey
    cured and processed, 43
    organically raised, 85
    3:1 vegetable-to-meat ratio, 64, 84, 93
Meatballs, Herb-Scented, 146–47
microbiome. *See* gut microbiome and digestive health
mineral broths
    in detox, 58–59
    Fish Stock, 175
    Mineral-Rich Bone Broth, 176
    Roasted Vegetable Stock, 174
mineral spray (Wild Mediterranean Sea Spray), 202
Mom's Secret Tzatziki, 177
Moussaka, 150–51
Myconian-Inspired Black-Eyed Peas, 128, *129*

N
Not-Your-Typical Greek Salad, 110, *111*
nuts and seeds
    Baklava Butter, *180*, 181
    Catalan Gazpacho, 109
    Chocolate Yogurt Sundae, 179
    in detox, 56
    Endive Salad from Beaune, 102, *103*
    Fresh Salad, 73
    Grapefruit Salad, 101
    Not-Your-Typical Greek Salad, 110, *111*
    Roasted Squash Seeds with Sea Salt, 127
    "Root-Down" Salad, *106*, 107

O
olive oil, 55–56, 88
"Olive Your Hair" Serum, 206

P
Paella, Jackson Pollock's, *132*, 133–34
Peppermint and Chamomile Tea, 73
personal care products
    Dried Fig and Coffee Exfoliant, 205
    "Honey, I'm Hot" Exfoliant, 205
    "Olive Your Hair" Serum, 206
    Tuscan Aromatic Room Spray, 202
    Wild Mediterranean Sea Spray, 202
    Yiayia's Horta Toner, 206
Pizza à la Stella, 137
poultry. *See* chicken; turkey
prebiotic and probiotic foods, 47, 48, 59, 60–61
probiotic and prebiotic foods, 47, 48, 59, 60–61
protein, 49, 64, 84–86
Provençal-Style Rub, 158
Provençal-Style Sole, 167

R
Rigatoni with Butternut Squash and Basil, 130–31
Risotto Classico, 136
Roast Chicken: Four Countries, Four Ways, *156*,
    157–58
Roasted Squash Seeds with Sea Salt, 127
Roasted Vegetable Stock, 174
Room Spray, Tuscan Aromatic, 202
"Root-Down" Salad, *106*, 107
rubs for roast chicken, 158

S
salads
    Berry and Chicken Salad, 73
    Endive Salad from Beaune, 102, *103*
    French-Meets-Greek Salad, 104
    Fresh Salad, 73
    Grapefruit Salad, 101
    Italian-Style Bean Salad, 123
    Lucca-Style Salad, 105
    Not-Your-Typical Greek Salad, 110, *111*
    "Root-Down" Salad, *106*, 107
sausage
    Jackson Pollock's Paella, *132*, 133–34
    Spanish-Style Baked Beans, 122

Scallop Skewers, Sweet, 170, *171*
sea-based main dishes. *See* fish and shellfish
Sea Bass, Greek-Style, 167
seafood. *See* fish and shellfish
sea salt, 60, 89
seasoning rubs for roast chicken, 158
Sea Spray, Wild Mediterranean, 202
sea-tox. *See* land-tox/sea-tox
sea vegetables, 58, 68, 121
seeds. *See* nuts and seeds
shellfish. *See* fish and shellfish
skin-care products. *See* personal care products
Sole, Provençal-Style, 167
soups
   Catalan Gazpacho, 109
   Everyone's Fish Stew, *168*, 169
   Fish Stock, 175
   Italian-Style Turkey 'n' Onion Soup, 74
   Mineral-Rich Bone Broth, 176
   Roasted Vegetable Stock, 174
   Rustic Vegetable Soup, 75
   St. Barts–Style Chilled Pea Soup, 112
Spanish-Style Baked Beans, 122
Spanish-Style Braised Beef, 163
Spanish-Style Rub, 158
Spinach Pie with Sprouted Wheat Crust, 118–19
Sprouted Cinnamon-Maple French Toast, 99
Sprouted "Crepes," 97
Sprouted Wheat Crust, Spinach Pie with, 118–19
Squash Seeds with Sea Salt, Roasted, 127
St. Barts–Style Chilled Pea Soup, 112
staple recipes
   Fish Stock, 175
   Mineral-Rich Bone Broth, 176
   Mom's Secret Tzatziki, 177
   Roasted Vegetable Stock, 174
   Wild Vinaigrette, 173
Steamed Vegetables, 74
Stew, Everyone's Fish, *168*, 169
stocks and broths
   in detox, 58–59
   Fish Stock, 175
   Mineral-Rich Bone Broth, 176
   Roasted Vegetable Stock, 174
stress management, 184, 190–97
Stuffed Sweet Potato, 74
Stuffed Zucchini, From-the-Village, *140*, 141–42

Sunchoke Chips, 108
Sundae, Chocolate Yogurt, 179
supplements
   for detox, 45–49
   HCL, 30, 53
   for land-tox/sea-tox, 68
   probiotics, 47
sweets
   Baklava Butter, *180*, 181
   Chocolate Yogurt Sundae, 179
Sweet Scallop Skewers, 170, *171*

T
tea
   Peppermint and Chamomile Tea, 73
   in Wild Mediterranean diet, 89–90
Toner, Yiayia's Horta, 206
Tonic, Lavender Lemonade, 73
topical mineral spray (Wild Mediterranean Sea Spray), 202
turkey
   Braised Turkey Breast, 154–55
   in detox, 56
   From-the-Village Stuffed Zucchini, *140*, 141–42
   Herb-Scented Meatballs, 146–47
   Italian-Style Turkey 'n' Onion Soup, 74
   sausage, *in* Spanish-Style Baked Beans, 122
   Stuffed Sweet Potato, 74
Tuscan Aromatic Room Spray, 202
Tzatziki, California-Style Homemade Gyro with Sprouted Tortilla and, 139
Tzatziki, Mom's Secret, 177

V
vegetables. *See also* beans and legumes; greens
   Briam, *114*, 115–16
   Burger with Whipped Potatoes, *152*, 153
   Catalan Gazpacho, 109
   daily servings, 63–64
   Deep-Dish Frittata, 95
   in detox, 55, 59–60
   Everyone's Fish Stew, *168*, 169
   Fava with Roasted Vegetables, *124*, 125–26
   fermented, 59
   From-the-Village Stuffed Zucchini, *140*, 141–42
   Moussaka, 150–51
   options, 81

to purchase, 80
Rigatoni with Butternut Squash and Basil,
   130–31
Roasted Vegetable Stock, 174
Rustic Vegetable Soup, 70
sea vegetables, 58, 68, 121
St. Barts–Style Chilled Pea Soup, 112
Steamed Vegetables, 74
Stuffed Sweet Potato, 74
Sunchoke Chips, 108
3:1 vegetable-to-meat ratio, 64, 84, 93
Vinaigrette, Wild, 173

W

Wild Detox
   caffeine during, 50
   diagnostic tests, 51–53
   foods for, 43–45, 54–61
   frequently asked questions, 77
   immunogenic foods, 44, 76
   meal guidelines, 63–64
   pre-detox self-test, 41
   purpose and components of, 33–34, 40–41
   recipes, 73–75
   sample regimen, 65
   to schedule, 42–43
   supplements, 45–49
   tips for success, 71
   transition back to lifelong style of eating, 41–42
Wild Detox land-tox/sea-tox
   customization for specific needs, 34, 40, 67
   foods for, 54–60

intermittent fasting, 66
   sample regimen, 65
   supplements, 68
Wild Mediterranean diet
   cost of, 89
   drinks, 89–90
   pantry, fridge, and freezer items, 86–88
   plant foods, 79–84
   proteins, 84–86
   3:1 vegetable-to-meat ratio, 64, 84, 93
   "village-to-table" approach, 42, 79, 93
Wild Mediterranean lifestyle
   alcohol consumption, 198–99
   childlike perspective, 184–85
   community and social relationships, 90–91, 183,
     198–99
   fun and exercise, 185–89
   joy and satisfaction, 183
   sleep, 197–98
   stress management, 184, 190–97
   website for support and advice, 208
Wild Mediterranean Sea Spray, 202
Wild Vinaigrette, 173

Y

Yiayia's Eggs Mati, 96
yogurt
   Chocolate Yogurt Sundae, 179
   Mom's Secret Tzatziki, 177
   Moussaka, 150–51
   as probiotic, 47
   St. Barts–Style Chilled Pea Soup, 112

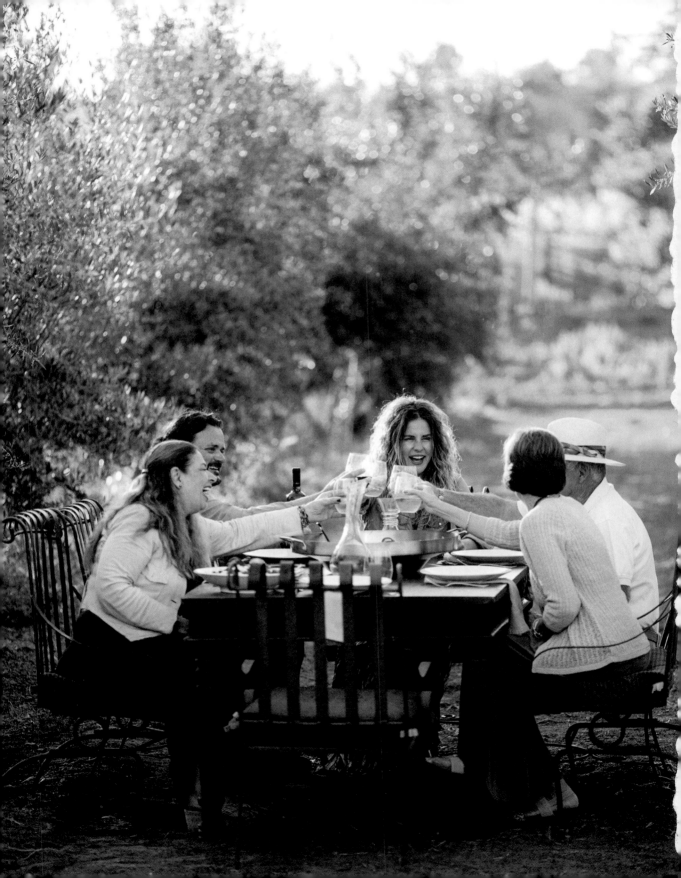